# LIFE AFTER HEART SURGERY

## DAVID A. BURKE

**Outskirts Press, Inc.**
**Denver, Colorado**

Outskirts Press, Inc.
http://www.outskirtspress.com

ISBN: 978-1-4327-3142-7

Outskirts Press and the "OP" logo are trademarks belonging to Outskirts Press, Inc.

PRINTED IN THE UNITED STATES OF AMERICA

# TABLE OF CONTENTS

# DEDICATION

This book is dedicated to Edwin S. Burke, my father. Ed or Whitey, as his friends called him because of his white hair, was born Aug 18, 1918 and died in the summer of 1975. He left behind his wife Virginia and his three boys, Jeff, Phillip and me. He was a dedicated father, devoted husband, semi-pro baseball player and worked very hard all his life.

# PREFACE

All patients do not respond to surgery exactly the same. Everyone is different, and the recovery will be a little different as well. You may have coronary artery bypass, stents or angioplasty for clogging, narrow or leaky valves, valve replacement or repair, or a combination of these. Some things remain the same, despite the differences. You may have had or are scheduled for stents or a heart replacement, a bypass, or something in between. This book is written in an attempt to help you understand how your life may change due to your surgery, and hopefully provide some insight for your family of what you are going through, as well as what they will go through with you.

# BACKGROUND ON THE AUTHOR

This is my story:

I will start my background with my father. Heredity, what is in your family genes, is a crucial factor. If heart disease is in your family history, then I'm afraid you have one strike against you, before you ever get up to the plate. My father's heart, while doomed to failure at the age of 57, was one of the biggest that I have ever had the pleasure to encounter. He served in the US army, worked two jobs and raised his three boys to be respectful of others. He was a soft-spoken man who would give you the shirt off his back and do anything for anyone. Everyone that knew him liked him and spoke fondly of him. He left us way too early and I love all the memories I have of him.

Now for me, I have had two open heart bypass surgeries, then a third chest opening surgery to remove two liters of fluid before I was 50 years old. Except for my family's names, I will leave out the names of the others in this story, to protect their privacy.

My first surgery was in October of 1989, at the age of 36. With a family history of heart trouble, it was not a surprise, it was a reality. I had planned for this inevitable surgery ever since my father died. This may sound strange, but I have always believed "forewarned is forearmed." I knew I had a heart like Dad, and that wasn't going to change. I never felt sorry for myself or "Woe is me." I simply made it part of my life and planned to be ready for whatever came my way. Working out daily was part of it.

My father, Ed, died of a massive heart attack when he was 57 years young. His father, Hugo, my grandfather, died of a heart attack at the age of 72. I only knew Grandfather as a small pre-school age child, before we lost him. I do remember hanging from his outstretched massive arms in failed attempts to pull them down. He was a powerful man. My grandfather on my mother's side was already gone, dying of heart trouble in his fifties as well. So I grew up with no grandfathers and lost my dad when I was 22. It has been a long time without him, and I feel so bad that he didn't get to know his grandchildren, and, now, great-grandchildren.

I grew up with a mitral valve prolapse, which caused chest pains ever since I was a teenager in high school. With this family history, I was told by many physicians that my competing in three varsity sports and living an active life consisting of many workouts would strengthen, enlarge and better my chances of having healthy arteries, and would help in recovery when heart surgery finally took place.

The mitral valve prolapse condition is when the valve does not close tightly enough after the chamber of the heart has filled with blood. When the heart beats, a small portion of the blood goes back out the valve, in the wrong direction, and causes a back pressure of blood against the blood that is ready to fill the heart again for the next heart beat. This backpressure causes a pain in your chest area that can drop you to your knees. There were many times that I would clutch my chest and fold forward from the resulting pain. This never occurred during all the sports activities that I was in. It always seemed to be while I was at rest. When they did occur, if I sat down or laid down, that usually helped it to subside and in a few minutes, I felt nothing.

In the ninth grade and very into athletics, I was hospitalized for surgery to remove a tumor on my right kidney, which the doctors found as a result of a routine physical because my blood pressure was high. It was 210/130, and high enough that the doctors admitted me into the hospital to find out why. The tumor was removed and I was left with a blood pressure of 150/100. I competed in cross country, basketball, and track and field throughout high school, and later ran the Decathlon for Central Michigan University, and even held the Javelin record for a short time for CMU. I started teaching right out of College in 1975. I continued in Decathlon competition and lifting and included a marathon, just so I could say: "I've done that."

In the 1971-72 school year, which was my freshman year at CMU, the lottery draft was still in use for the United States Military, and the Vietnam War was just concluding. My lottery draft number was 26, which meant I was to report to Detroit for my physical. In those days, every birth date was assigned a number, drawn at random, and anyone whose birthday had a number of 125 and under was heading into the military. "I was heading into the service."

While in Detroit for my physical, the military learned that my blood pressure was higher than their acceptable standards. I was tested many times over the next few days and was rejected from Military Service because of the high blood pressure, which was 170/105 in the final test. It was a tense time.

I am very patriotic and was willing to accept my responsibility to serve for this great country. My father, as I mentioned, was in the Army, and my oldest brother was in the Marine Corp Reserves; and while I was scared, I was ready. I've always stood and paid tribute to our flag when our National Anthem is played. I have a little trouble with those who do not pay their respect, but understand their right in not wanting to. With that said, it still bothers me if they are not at least quiet during the national anthem and don't respect the people around them and their right to stand and pay tribute. I now have a son-in-law who is a former Marine, and re-enlisted into the Army, Special Forces, and I am very proud of him and of his service to the country.

I graduated CMU in 1975 with a BS in Education and began teaching and coaching immediately in Small-town, USA in the fall of 1975. I continued to work out and compete in road races, AAU decathlons and lifting weights. I was also coaching the age group swim team, varsity cross country, varsity track and field and then added varsity volleyball, a year later, to the list. Seven years later, while still teaching, I opened health clubs and began coaching and competing in power lifting which I continued for 10 years until my first open heart surgery.

You need to know, if you haven't figured it out already, I am the eternal optimist. The cup is always half full, and never half empty. I have had, to date, three knee surgeries, two lower back surgeries, two shoulder surgeries, elbow surgery, kidney surgery, hernia, a growth in my neck, and two open heart surgeries and a third into the chest to remove two liters of fluid. That's over a dozen, if you're counting and I still look for the positive, and plan how to recover and get back in shape afterwards. Each surgery, I go into like an athletic contest that I prepare for, by being in shape and start thinking of recovery exercises and what I can do, even before the surgery takes place. When I started writing this book, I was recovering from right shoulder surgery for the second time, for complete re-attachment of the rotator cuff and a torn bicep tendon. I recovered nicely from that surgery and returned to the weight room and or course pushed it too hard and will have surgery on my left shoulder by the time this book goes to print in the summer of 2008. And you know it. I have already contacted the Health Club where I train, and set up a two week freeze on my membership, and then I will be back in there with continued training.

With my family history, I had the knowledge that heart surgery was eminent, but I was the youngest of three boys in my family, full of energy, and wanted to be in a sport all the time. In the summer time, I would run and lift weights, swim, and practice my basketball shot every day, to stay ready for the next sport to start. Going to school was something I had to do, before I would be able to go to practice for the sport of the season. The summer before my high school senior year, my running workouts were 10 miles per day and I was always back to the house in less than an hour.

My doctors along the way had informed me that working out would probably make all the arteries around the heart and in my body stronger and enhance recovery in my eventual surgery. So, I worked hard and played hard all my life and never held back because of the heredity pool I was in. Staying in shape was what I wanted and now it had even more meaning for me.

I was married with three wonderful kids by the time my chest pains had increased to the point that I could not work out for more than five minutes before pains would force me to sit down, yet I still tried. I never said anything to the kids about it. They were one, five and nine years old at the time, and just needed to be kids.

I went to my local doctor and said: "Doc, I am ready for heart surgery." He didn't believe in my analysis, so he checked my vitals and so on. He didn't really believe it and thought I was crazy. He said, "There are a few things we need to check first." I said, "I know we will have to jump through all the hoops first and take all the tests required before surgery, but I know my body and my family history and I can tell you that it's time." He was still a little skeptical and not moving as fast as I knew we had too, so I insisted on scheduling a treadmill test quickly. He set me up with a cardiologist for the Bruce Protocol treadmill test.

## Treadmill Test

The treadmill test was the following week and again, it was an athletic test for me, but I knew what was going to happen. I was on the treadmill for less than four minutes before the pains started and their EKG leads were showing a problem as well. I went into the very painful category very quickly and Doc shut the test down. I was standing by the treadmill and given a nitro tablet and told to lie down. I said to the Doctor. "Doc, I've been running and coaching for a long time, and you never lie down immediately after running." I stand 6'2", at 210 pounds, and the 5'4" doctor got on his toes and in my face and in a stronger tone, said, "I said, Lie down." So I did. The nitro calmed things down in my heart, by opening the arteries and allowing better blood flow, and we scheduled the next test, which was a heart catherization. With the use of the nitro, I experienced pressure in the back of my head, in the lower quadrant and the chest pains subsided within minutes.

Nitroglycerin (nitro) can widen or dilate the arteries and improve blood flow to your heart. Nitro can be given through a skin patch, pills, an ointment, or a spray. This medicine may also be used to relieve angina pain.

We scheduled a heart catheterization that was done within a few days and the results were again what I expected. I was scheduled for bypass surgery. The test revealed 3 arteries were 99% blocked, one was 75% and another was 50% blocked. I was scheduled for bypass surgery with a great surgeon in Grand Rapids, who is now retired. I was to be the youngest patient at the age of 36, scheduled for bypass in that hospital at that time in 1989.

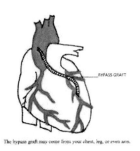

The bypass graft may come from your chest, leg, or even arm.

Bypass surgery is the most common type of heart surgery, with more than hundreds of thousand successful bypass surgeries in the United States each year. Bypass surgery improves the blood flow to the heart with a new route, or "bypass" around the section of clogged or diseased artery. The surgery involves sewing a section of vein from the leg or artery from the chest or another part of the body to bypass the part of the diseased coronary artery. This creates a new route for blood to flow, so that the heart muscle will get the oxygen-rich blood it needs to work property.

Coronary artery disease (CAD) affects almost 1.3 million Americans, making it the most common form of heart disease. CAD and its complications, like arrhythmia, angina pectoris, and heart attack (also called myocardial infarction), are the leading causes of death in the United States. CAD most often results from a condition known as arteriosclerosis, which happens when a waxy substance forms inside the arteries that supply blood to your heart. This substance, called plaque, is made of cholesterol, fatty compounds, calcium, and a blood clotting material called fibrin.

## Listening To Your Body

This is so important. Many people, especially men, do not go to see the doctor when they should. They may feel a slight pain, or get dizzy occasionally, feel short of breath and pass it off as anything other than a clue that there is a problem with their heart. Men tend to work through pain, push through, and have been taught that their whole life: "Don't whine," "Don't be a baby," "Suck it up," and so on. With this type of background, it is difficult to then say to yourself or your spouse, I think I need some help until it is so bad that by the time they go in, they may need the surgery already. I am now an advocate to others to get to your Doctor and check. I have always been very good about what I call "Listen to your body." I have used it for myself and with all the athletes I have ever coached. Please don't misconstrue my former statement about men tending to work through pain. I am not saying men are tougher than women, but I am saying boys are raised to not be a wuss, but to tough it out. Right or wrong is a different debate, but it is what our culture does.

# CHAPTER 1

## * Waiting For Heart Surgery Date

My surgery was scheduled with a waiting period of almost two weeks. Surgery would take place in Grand Rapids, Michigan, very close to where I grew up and where my mother and step Dad still live. At the time, I was the youngest patient that this hospital had ever performed an open heart bypass surgery on. When talking to the doctor, I told him my story and history and that I fully expected to get back to full recovery and to do it quickly. Even though I knew heart surgery was coming, there still was not a good time to be laid up and take recovery time and so on, in my busy schedule. So I just wanted to; "get it done" and get back to my life. I was still a full time teacher and owned two health clubs and coached a power lifting team as well as competing myself in power lifting.

The two week wait was a very anxious time. I look at surgeries like one would plan for an athletic event where I prepare mentally and then I am ready to go. Some of you remember the movie, Brian's Song, which inspired me. I prepared and was ready and then the waiting period felt like an eternity. I continued to go to the gym and as the surgery got closer, and I continued to work out and finally got cautious. I thought, how stupid to work out now and have a heart attack and blow it when I knew surgery was scheduled next week, so I went home and let the workouts go until after surgery. While I had a lot of confidence in the surgeon in Grand Rapids, I did a lot of praying and asking for God to guide the good doctor throughout the surgery. I did hang onto the knowledge that being in better shape would make the recovery time quicker and easier.

It was now 1989, and every year that passed since my father passed away, I knew that heart surgery was inevitable for me. I took confidence that the medical profession was getting better and better at this open heart surgery procedure.

Your operation will usually be scheduled at a time that is best for you and your surgeon, except in urgent cases. As the date of your surgery gets closer, be sure to tell your surgeon and cardiologist about any changes in your health. If you have a cold or the flu, this can lead to infections that may affect your recovery. Be aware of fever, chills, coughing, or a runny nose. Tell the doctor if you have any of these symptoms. You will need to have a list of any medicines you are taking. Your doctor will ask for it, and more than likely will instruct you when to stop or continue your medication.

## Zipper Club

This Club is made up of all the patients who have had their chests cracked open. Sorry if that description scares you, but that is what I have heard, even from medical personnel, when referring to going inside the chest for an open heart surgery. When a patient goes through an open heart surgery, the result will be a scar down the sternum of the chest of about five to nine inches in length, usually with three drainage tube scars on the upper abdominal muscles. You are now in the zipper club. People are not knocking the door down to get into this club. However, if you are in need of open heart surgery, the alternative to getting into the club is far worse.

I designed a shirt and wear it proudly. I minored in art in college, and am a collector of ideas to create my own. The design shown above is what I came up with. I sold a few of the shirts, after the first surgery. I currently have a website of online clothing which is "Sportswear for Success" or SUCwear, and you can find the zipper club shirt there. Go to www.sucwear.com. At the time of this publication, the site was under construction.

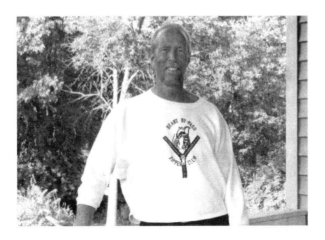

## While On Heart Surgery Waiting List

Allow me to go back in history briefly. In 1975, my father at age 57 was having heart trouble. He went in and had the heart catheterization and they found blockage in arteries in his heart. Open heart surgery was a relatively new procedure in those days. My father's condition was viewed as not as much of an emergency as others to be scheduled for surgery. It was decided to treat my father with medication, in an attempt to dissolve the clogs. Within a week, he was doing things that he was doing before, had returned to work, was doing odd jobs around the house and about a month later returned to golf, which he loved very much.

I remember during this time frame, summer time, my new wife of 6 months and I had moved near Mom and Dad's and we were around a lot, as not only did I enjoy the pool at their house, I helped them take care of it. I felt like we had to tie Dad down because he wanted to get back and do everything he always did right away. We all kept telling him to relax and just sit and recover from the tests and the fact that he had gone in to check what was wrong and he needed to slow down. He had to be doing something all the time. I took the push broom from him many times as he felt he should sweep the deck around the pool, the grass needed to be cut or something. He always held down two jobs and I don't ever remember him just sitting and doing nothing. We felt like Dad had gotten the message to take it slow, but it was tough for him.

We were at Mom and Dad's house to take a dip in the pool, on a hot summer day in Michigan. Dad returned from a golf game that he was telling us about where he had shot a pretty good round. It felt good that Dad was back to normal activities for him and he was generally pretty quiet and never boastful about himself. I had asked him to tell me about his round that day, so he told me about it and he seemed very happy.

The main quote from my Father that I would like to share that I have cherished and passed on to others, including my kids is, "You don't ever have to talk about yourself, or brag. If you are as good as you think you are, then the people will know it already. On the other hand, if you have to tell them how good you are, then you are not as good as you think you are, or they would have known it already." Whenever I shared this quote with others, including many athletes I have coached, I would preface it with, "A wise Ol' Man told me once," then I would deliver his statement.

Mom and Dad had a poodle, because it was the only kind of dog Dad wasn't allergic too, but the little rascal would leave messes on the floor, so during the day, he was kept downstairs where there was a linoleum floor. At this point, Dad then went downstairs to check if there was any mess to attend to, when my wife heard a strange guttural groan from the basement. She called to me immediately saying. "Dave, you better go check on Dad." That was a scary sound from down there. I ran to him only hitting one step of the 13 on the way down.

I found him on the floor, on his side, lifeless. I rolled him to his back and felt a fast pulse at the wrist. I had just finished a CPR training class and had some knowledge of first aid. I then checked his breathing and he was not breathing on his own. I immediately started mouth-to-mouth and called upstairs to my wife to call for an ambulance. By this time only 30 seconds had elapsed, and I continued mouth to mouth. My wife called for an ambulance and then came downstairs and then went back upstairs to go outside to direct the paramedics inside.

The ambulance and paramedics arrived within six minutes of the call and came downstairs where Dad and I were. Those six minutes were the longest minutes of my life. My Dad was on his back, lifeless, and I was blowing life into him hoping and praying the whole time that it was working. The paramedics did their evaluation of Dad and my method of providing mouth-to-mouth for him. They told me to continue, which helped answer my internal question of, Was I doing it correctly? They started CPR, and timed their compressions with my breathing, and they started their count of compressions and then instructed me to blow. They moved Dad to a gurney, and set up an automatic CPR and breathing machine that was hooked to the side of the bed and took over the CPR and breathing process. This allowed them to carry him upstairs and the CPR continued right into the ambulance. The fact that they started chest compression worried me, as I had felt a pulse. Could I have been wrong about the pulse?

My mother arrived home just as we were getting Dad into the ambulance and I jumped in the car with her. She had to approach the house and see the ambulance and police car lights flashing in her own driveway and had that awful sinking feeling that it was her husband. Mom and I followed the ambulance to the hospital. We were there in less than 10 minutes and we were still within 30 minutes of the time Dad went down. Other family members were called and met us at the hospital and we all waited for news.

About 20 minutes later, a doctor came and informed us that Dad was gone. In his autopsy, they discovered he suffered a massive heart attack and probably died instantly. The doctor said that the pulse I felt at the wrist was more than likely a fibulation of the heart after the attack. where it beats quickly for a few moments after heart attack. Because I had gotten to him so fast, that was still going on.

Dad left us way too early. I was only 22 years old, and he had just gotten his third and final son through college. I thank God he was able to see that and make my wedding 6 months before, and he was there for my final collegiate decathlon competition in the MAC for CMU. In high school, my parents never missed an athletic event that my brothers and I were in. When I competed in College in the Decathlon, I know it was tough on Dad to have to miss them. But we competed all over the country and it was impossible, plus the decathlon has 5 events on Friday and 5 on Saturday for a gruling event to compete and watch. He made plans to make my final competition for CMU my senior year just 2 months before he died. When I was done, he and I walked with an arm around each other one last lap around the track. I remarked to him, "This is the last competition I will ever do competing for someone else, for a school. Anything else I compete in will be just for me." And we walked a final lap together.

I'd like to say this about my Dad. He always kissed his boys on the lips from day one that we were born and until he died. When we saw each other or said goodbye, we would kiss and never question why. We loved him and he saw no reason that he could not kiss his boys and he taught that to us. There was only one time that I turned my head, when he dropped me off to college and there were others around and I felt self-conscious about it. He never said anything, but I felt so bad that I had done that, I had to wait two hours for them to get back home, so I could call him and apologize and tell him again that I loved him. I never turned my head again, and my son kisses his Dad too, without ever a thought of anyone's opinion.

I think of Dad often.I'm 55 now, and my youngest, my son is 22 years old and graduated college in 2008. My son and I are similar ages to when my Dad passed away 33 years ago. I want to be around longer into his life than my Dad was into mine. Dad has been gone for so many years and I have missed having him in my life, and feel badly that he had to miss his kids' lives.

Just from my family, he missed my first daughter being born, her greatness, her athletics, her college volleyball scholarship, marriage, and birth of his great-granddaughter. My second daughter, the singer, the athlete, her earning 1st team All-State in two different sports in high school, her college full ride basketball scholarship, earning Patriot League tournament most valuable player, and moving on to be the youngest female to be hired as Women's director of Basketball at a Big 10 school, and the first in the family to get her Masters degree.. My third child, my son, who became such a gentleman and was a three-sport high school athlete with school records in track in the sprints, and football All-State, as well and a full ride football collegiate scholarship as a wide receiver and then earning All-league honors there. Just recently, he has passed his DAT's and is ready for Dental School.

My second marriage and meeting my wife, and her youngest daughter who was the matchmaker for me and her Mom. She became my stepdaughter, and later I adopted her and she went on to also earn a collegiate scholarship and became a Physical Therapy Assistant. Even though Dad missed all these events, I am a believer that there is a heaven and Dad is there and somehow he is watching over us and knows all these wonderful things already.

I am proud of all of my children and want to be here as long as possible to share in their lives. My adopted daughter never met her dad as he had died a month before she was born, so I don't want her to lose another one too soon. I have already been able to give my oldest daughter away at her wedding, to her husband, witness their wedding and deliver a speech about them at their reception. I was there when their beautiful baby girl was born, my glorious granddaughter. I was at my second daughter's college basketball games and her graduation and I have visited her at her new job, have been able to watch all my son's games through college and watch him graduate college as well, and listen to him play the guitar and sing as well. These are the things my Dad had to miss, and that makes me sad.

# CHAPTER 2

## Heart Bypass Surgery Time

Most patients are admitted to the hospital the day before surgery, or in the morning of an afternoon scheduled surgery. You will be asked to bath or shower to reduce germs on your skin. Upon reporting into the hospital for surgery, physically, I did not look like the typical heart surgery patient. I was only 36 years old, tipping the scales at 210, after training for power lifting for 10 years and I could successfully perform lifts of a 545 pound full squat, a 380 pound pause bench-press and a 580 pound dead lift, with 7% body fat. I entered the hospital at 205 pounds by surgery date, already having lost 5 pounds from backing off on my training, for two weeks.

Going into my surgery, I never felt scared. I had faith in the surgeon and the medical staff and faith in God as well. Even if the surgery didn't leave me in this world, I was content with the fact that I knew I was going to be able to be reunited with my Dad. He was a good man and I knew he was in heaven ready to embrace me as well. I did learn that my surgeon had performed 240 of these surgeries the year before mine and that gave me even more confidence as I realized that to him, fixing another heart was like playing with tinker toys. I felt that I was in good hands, and went in with an attitude of "Let's get this done so I can get back to my life." I am an optimist as

I have stated, even though my world was crashing down around me.

My life had gone from great to bad in a quick hurry, as my wife and I were separated at the time, and the stress was not a good ingredient to add to this already, poor, inherited trait of clogged arteries. No blame intended for the stress, this surgery was inevitable. Other things would eventually occur in this year that just added up to a year that would be good to forget.

My friend and minister from my church went to the hospital with me to drop me off. Rev. and I, after checking in went into the room assigned, and were sitting in the two lounge chairs provided, next to the bed. We were sitting there talking when a nurse came in and said, "Mr. Burke?" I observed immediately that she didn't know who was who when she glanced back and forth at the Rev and me, so I took that opportunity to point to the Rev. He protested right away that it wasn't him, and I said, "Come on, Dave, let the nurse do her job and stop fooling around." The nurse then addressed him as Mr. Burke and started her questions of him. He protested again and scampered from his chair to his feet, as she wanted him to change into his hospital gown. He protested some more and was getting quite nervous that she thought he was me, and he started digging for his wallet for his license, so I finally admitted that I was Mr. Burke. She giggled and then directed her instructions to me and I showed her the hospital bracelet that the desk had put on me and we proceeded with the check-in procedure and putting on the hospital gown, that was open back (what ever that was, that covered nothing). We laughed about that later, but at the time, the Rev. didn't think it was very funny. His blood pressure went way up in that few moments. If he ever reads this, he will smile again.

I then received all the visits from the nurses with shaving preparation, the anesthesiologist informing me of what his procedure would be and the surgeon with comments and time for any final questions before surgery, scheduled for the following day.

My mother was there when it was time to go into a briefing room that night before surgery for about five patients who were all scheduled for heart surgery. The room quieted down when the presenter, who was ready to start a video said, "We'll get started as soon as Mr. Burke arrives." I said: "You've got him, go ahead and roll it." We all waited for about five more minutes in silence and people stared to talk to each other again. So I asked quietly first to my mom about what are we waiting for, and she said I don't know. I finally asked the presenter: "What are we waiting for?" Then, he answered: "We have to wait for Mr. Burke to get started; they are checking his room now for him." I explained more clearly: "I am Mr. Burke, the one scheduled for surgery, you can start the video." In disbelief, he started the program and we watched. My mom was 65 years old at the time, so the presenter thought I was the son of the patient and he had to wait for Mr. Burke to start the video. My mom and I laughed about that whole scene many times as well after surgery. As mentioned, I was the youngest bypass surgery patient that this hospital would perform at that time.

I don't know how the others felt about this explanation and video, as I never asked anyone, but for me, I could have done without it. It was designed to show the family what a heart patient would go through and how they would look after surgery, so the family wouldn't be too shocked when they saw the patient, bloated with extra fluid in them and a tube out of every possible orifice plus some manmade holes as well. This started chest pains in me as I probably over analyze everything, and I was watching intently. So I had to go back to a happy place and relax to calm down, as surgery was tomorrow for me.

I got my last visit with my first wife (kids and family, and was wheeled in. The anesthesiologist's needle was in place already, and all he would have to do is administer the medicine when the time came.

Prior to surgery, I said to the doctor, "God be with you in surgery and guide your hands." He said, "I'll see you afterwards."

Then the anesthesiologist started the medicine and said, "You're going off to sleep now, we'll see you in the recovery room." I felt the medicine move up my arm in about two seconds, it felt cold. By the time it hit my upper arm, and my shoulder area, I don't remember another thing. I was out for the surgery to begin.

Surgery went well, and after four hours, I emerged with five bypasses, three of which, they were able to use arteries from my chest and two from my left leg. All of the bypasses were on the back of the heart. The doctor said due to the fact that I had worked out so much, that the arteries in my chest were large enough that he could use three of them and still leave enough to feed my chest. They would rather use chest arteries, because, they are feeders already to the chest muscles and they only have to disconnect one end and redirect it past a clogged artery to feed that area of the heart. I had talked to the surgeon before the surgery, and requested that if they were going to take arteries from my leg, to start with my left leg, as I had a small varicose bulge just behind the left knee. So if they took arteries from that leg, they could eliminate that bulge at the same time. I also asked that if there were not enough artery pieces that they needed by the time they reached the knee, to go to the right leg and go up to the knee as well. I felt that I would rather have matching scars on each leg; instead of one scar all the way up on the left leg. Plus at that time, when they were still slicing you all the way up the leg with a full leg-long cut, I had heard that it is more painful up towards the top of the thigh, than it is in the lower leg. Now they do little dash cuts about every 6 inches apart up the leg.

I am a structured, organized, yes probably anal person, and I preferred matching leg scars. As it worked out, they only needed to get artery pieces up to the knee on my left leg. They took care of the varicose veins behind my knee and there was no pain. The doctor explained to everyone that had come in my support, how things went in surgery, and that he expected a good recovery based on how fit I was.

## Surgery Specifics

I was scheduled for morning surgery, so by 6:00 a.m., the nurses were in my room, with final preparation. My chest was shaved of the few sparse hairs that existed, and I was given the pre-surgery shot to help relax you. Some call it the "Happy Shot," which makes you sleepy. I remember joking with them about that. Why do you come into a room at 6:00 a.m. and wake me up to give me a shot to make me sleepy? They laughed and explained it was also to help the patient relax. An hour or so later, I said goodbye and see you soon to my Mom and stepfather, and they wheeled me off to surgery. I arrived in the operating room, and they moved me over onto the operating table. I remember the nurses saying, "Look at this guy, full of muscle and here for heart surgery." The Doctor said that they would be administering the anesthesia soon, and I would drift off to sleep and wake up in the Cardiac Intensive Care Unit, CICU. I drifted off to sleep just as he had said.

I mentioned my stepfather. He is a wonderful man that my mom met after Dad had passed away, and I call him Dad, because that is what he is to me. I felt I should explain that, if I mention Dad later in the book, you would know whom I was referring too. My biological Father had already passed away and I now call my stepfather: Dad. My mom has been married to him for over 30 years now, which is another testimonial to "Life after Heart Trouble", as Mom was left behind and found love again. Ever since I met my Dad, I knew he was a great guy and was so happy for my Mom and for him that they had found each other.

While asleep, you are hooked up to a respirator, a breathing tube is inserted into your throat towards the lungs and the respirator is breathing for you. They then make the cut on the skin over the sternum and then use a tool for cutting the sternum. I'm told the tool which cuts through the sternum very easily, has a little flat foot on the end of it which they guide just under the sternum from bottom to top and cut the sternum; in simple terms, it is like an electric knife. The sternum is then clamped apart at a distance that the surgeon could gain easy access to do his job. This clamping of the sternum apart stresses the ribs apart, flexes them all the way to your back where they are connected to your backbone. A patient sometimes feels discomfort in their back and this is why.

Next, the surgeon has to cut into and remove the pericardium, which is a sack of fluid that the heart is suspended in and floats within giving it a final line of defense against a blunt hit, or hard blow to the chest and torso, and the fluid helps cushion the heart in the blow, like a car crash. This sack is not replaced, it is irreparable and a person can and does survive without it. One thing that is necessary during surgery is the use of the iron lung. This machine is hooked up to you to keep the blood flowing through your body during surgery, when they disconnect your heart to work on it. When they do this, 2/3 of your blood is removed and saved and replaced with a saline solution, so that it is thinner and will go through the machine easier. Now, the iron lung is feeding the body and brain, and has replaced the heart for the time during surgery and keeps the blood oxygenated and flowing throughout the body during surgery. Your heart is stopped from beating and they are ready to work on it. In my case, they were prepared to perform a 5-way bypass, or fix five clogged arteries, all of which, I was told, were in the back of my heart.

Now let's make sure that you understand what happens in a bypass. Example: You have a 99% blockage in artery A in the back of the heart and the clog is about 1/4'" long. A bypass would be a vein taken from the leg or arm and sewn onto artery A before and after the blockage, looking like an exit ramp loop of a highway. The new bypass carries the blood around the blocked portion of the artery and feeds the area of the heart that is meant to be fed by that clogged artery.

They were able to use three mammary arteries in my case. This was due to the fact that I had worked out hard for many, many years and the auxiliary capillaries in my chest were large enough to keep my chest muscle fed with blood after they redirected the mammary arteries for the bypasses. When using these arteries, they only have to disconnect one end of the mammary artery and pull it past the blockage and connect, again making a new feeder for that part of the heart past the clog. This process was done for three blocked arteries. They then used veins from my left leg for the other two clogged arteries. As planned earlier, they took the needed bypass material from my leg and when they got to the inside back of my knee, they removed the small cluster of varicose veins that I had in that area. They did not need to go any higher than my knee with the leg cut. After the three mammary arteries were used, two more bypasses were repaired and it was time to hook me back up. Next it is time to place in the drainage tubes. These three tubes are placed one around each lung and the last around the heart to carry any fluids and excess drainage from the surgery area out of the body. They then reconnect the heart to the body and disconnect from the iron lung. The surgical staff then starts to put your blood back into you that was removed earlier. The addition of your own blood back into your body can make a patient look bloated. Remember, there was a need to add saline solution so your blood would pass through the iron lung easier.

The extra fluid will be eliminated through urinating, and absorption into the body. The three drainage tubes in layman's terms are like weep tile and will give the extra fluids from around the heart and lungs after surgery a way to drain out. These three tubes, about the size of a magic marker in circumference, come out of three holes made for them in your upper abdominal area. The three tubes in this surgery then merged into one tube and extended to a fluid collection chamber that was on the floor next to me. They then place the heart back into the body properly and release the clamps holding your sternum apart and prepare to connect the two sides together. Small holes are drilled on both sides of the cut sternum and small wires are placed through the holes and wrapped to hold the sternum tight together. This is done in about four places down the sternum. The skin is then sutured or stapled, bandaged and you are ready for CICU.

## The Recovery Room

I awoke in CICU still medicated, so I was in and out, but I remember there was still a tube down my throat and I could not talk yet. This was still part of the respirator needed to keep me breathing through surgery and I'm told that your body is not quite ready to take over breathing on its own right away, so the tube is still necessary for a little while. A nurse was right there and I was able to make hand signals pointing at the tube and a motion with my thumb towards the ceiling, meaning take this out. The nurse consoled me with the knowledge that she understood I wanted it out, but it had to stay in for another 30 minutes. That time past quickly; as I said, you are still medicated and you are in and out of consciousness. The respirator slid out without effort as the nurse pulled it and I could speak. Some patients will never be awake to experience this part. My voice was a little raspy for a couple days, again due to the tube down my throat.

Then people were able to visit me one or two at a time. My mom was there already. As I remember, I woke up with my hand in hers. I was in CICU for that day, and then I was brought back to my private room. I saw most of my family that day, but my kids were too young to see their Dad that day.

After surgery, the pericardium sack cannot be replaced. Because of that fact, you are prone to infection. Example: When getting your teeth cleaned at the dentist, there will be plaque released from between your teeth and you will have some bleeding. This could travel to your heart and cause a problem. So you need to take a pre-med prior to having the teeth work done. This is one of the things you learn afterwards, as there are just too many things to explain before surgery. That is the purpose of this book to help patients and family members to understand some of these things.

Next we will cover the days after surgery so you know what to expect. Everyone's rate of recovery will be different and now it is time to place your trust in your nurses and doctors to guide you through this stage towards recovery.

# CHAPTER 3

## What To Expect After Your Open Heart Surgery

This information is presented as a possible guide to help with questions that patients, families, and friends ask concerning the surgery. As well as what to expect in recovery, rehabilitation and life after heart surgery. It should be noted that if your doctor's instructions are different in any way than those talked about in this book, you should always follow the instructions of your doctor. They are familiar with you and your case. The information found within is based on my own experience, information gathered from my doctors and nurses, and talking to friends who have had heart surgery as well.

My goal was to get on the road to recovery ASAP. The first day after a short stint in CICU, I was back in my private room and the nurse came in and said we could go for a walk, and I was excited and ready to go for it. She brought in two other nurses as this process had more to it than I expected.

## Cardiac Rehabilitation

The first walk: The nurses raised the bed up to a sitting position and we swung my legs over to one side. Now it was time to get all the tubes and cords under control, the drainage tubes merged into one and entered into a monitoring/measuring box that was on the floor next to my bed. I learned quickly that this briefcase sized box had to be carried with me anywhere I moved. The intravenous tube had its own rolling tower. They helped me put on the slippers, and three nurses pulled and heaved until I was standing. Next, we paused in this standing position to make sure I wasn't dizzy. We started the walk and went about five baby steps, barely past the end of the bed, then turned around and went back. The process of tube and cord management in reverse, and I was back in bed. I felt like I had just run five miles so I then slept for about two and half hours. When I awoke, I was ready for some food and another walk.

My second walk was still difficult in terms of all the equipment going with me, but we managed to make it to the end of the bed and all the way to the private room door. It was probably 10 feet to the door, so I was pleased with the progress and improvement, but equally as happy to get back to the bed, as I was exhausted. My goal was just to walk farther each time I tried. Next time, we would go out into the hall.

By the second day, my recovery was going very well. I went for a walk in the morning around the cardiac wing that I was in, which had a small circuit, or loop, that would bring you back to where you started. It was a triangle circuit. The nurse was happy with making it out into the hall, but I insisted that we make the circuit. It was a challenge, but I made it and then slept hard again. I took two more walks that day around the circuit, much to the amazement of all the staff. In the next four days, I continued to increase the distance each time I went for a walk, two laps, three laps, four laps and then just started watching the clock and set a new goal of how many minutes I could walk.

I received great care from the hospital, and the food was tolerable. My brothers were there to visit me a lot and so were my kids; it was a joy to see them. My oldest daughter of 12 understood more about the procedure than my younger daughter of 8 and son of only 3 at the time. A couple of teacher friends made the trip to GR to visit as other family members did. It was good to see people as I felt like a caged animal compared to the level of activity I was used to.

I was dropping body weight like a brick, at a rate of four to five pounds per day. I was anxious to go home, but also apprehensive because I would be away from the constant watchful eye of the hospital. The large drainage tubes stayed in my chest until it was time to go home.

One day while still in the hospital, I told my Mother that there were two things I wanted to do before dying. And she said: "You're not going to die yet." But I went on to say, "I want to play basketball with my brother again, and I never jumped out of an airplane." She responded with. "You can play ball with your brother again if you want, but that idea of jumping out of an airplane is a stupid one." We both laughed. I had played on the same high school basketball team with my brother and wanted to play in the 3-on-3 Macker tournaments held around Michigan. So the next time my brother came up to see me, I asked him if he was willing to team up again and he said yes. He may have thought that I would forget about it, or wished I did. He was the better basketball player, and I knew we would be good with him playing. Later we did hook up for many 3-on-3 tournaments and even won one of them, and won the "Sportsmanship Award" in another. Much to my mother's dismay, I also jumped out of an airplane, which we'll talk about later.

While in the hospital, I broke all the norms on recovery, but the norms were written for an age bracket above mine, so they worked with me and let me set some new norms. Every day when I took my walks, I would add more and more laps around the circuit of the cardiac ward. All the nurses and doctors and patients got used to me being in the hall more than my room. I continued to take my walks throughout the night. I have always been a frequent flyer to the restroom during the night. So every time I had to go, I included a few laps of the circuit in the hall.

One thing that concerned me was when the surgeon said the following: 1. The veins that we use out of someone's leg only last about 10-12 years, and 2. All of your bypasses are on the back of your heart, and I hope I am retired by the time you need it again. I went home and still didn't know exactly what he meant. On the first part, about these veins lasting 10-12 years? What happens to them at that time, do they just blow up, rip out on the side, deteriorate, clog up like the original, or what? Then on the second statement: Did he mean, that it is such a mess in there, that he didn't want to be the one to have to go back in, or that he had done such a good job, that he would be retired before I needed a surgeon again. What I learned later was that they will clog again as the heredity situation did not change for me, and I also learned that the doctor did a great job on me.

## It's Perfectly Normal That

If an artery in your chest, called a mammary artery, was used, then you may feel some numbness to the left of your incision. Do not worry, this is normal.

If you have steri-strips on your incision, you may have to remove them, if they have not fallen off after about a week. Check with your doctor.

Your appetite will change. It may take a number of weeks before your appetite returns to the way it was. Some notice that their sense of taste is different, weaker or almost absent. Some will have nausea at just the smell of food for a few days to a couple weeks, but your normal appetite will return.

Many experience mood swings and feel depressed. Once again, you have just been through a lot and these feelings will come and go. Don't get discouraged, these feelings will disappear as well, and your improvement can be measured daily on how you feel and what you are able to do. I set goals and then start taking the steps to achieve those goals. I've always believed: "If you don't have a target, how are you going to hit it?"

Some will experience swelling in the legs, especially if you have one with an incision where they used veins. Elevating the legs will help and if the doctor gave you the compression socks, or elastic stockings, then use them.

Some have constipation problems for a couple reasons. Some pain medication may cause this, plus the urge to push is reduced after what you have been through. A laxative may work, but check with your doctor first. You may also add some fruits, fiber and juice to your diet to help as well.

You may have difficulty sleeping, or sleeping very long, or falling back to sleep after you wake up at night. This will improve also, and if you were prescribed pain pills, taking one before bed may help this. I experienced very little pain in my chest area. What was gone was the pain from the heart, so any discomfort from the incision was minimal.

You may actually notice clicking in your chest. This can occur for the first few days or even weeks after surgery but it should occur less and less as time goes on and be completely gone within a few weeks. Your sternum was cut in half, so let it heal.

You may experience muscle pain or tightness in your shoulders and upper back between the shoulder blades. Your pain medicine will help this, and as you start using these muscles more again, that feeling will improve.

You may get tired for the first couple of weeks, so when you have visitors and need to rest you will need to excuse yourself and go rest. Your visitors will understand. You need to use your energy for your physical therapy, which will get you back to independence sooner.

## Side Effects

Some medicines have side effects, so be aware of the possibility and be ready to call your doctor with questions. Some side effects may include nausea, diarrhea, constipation, stomach pain, vomiting, and dizziness, lightheadedness in standing, confusion, tingling in the hands and feet, extremely slow or fast pulse, bruising, skin rash. and others. Stay in communication with your doctor and/or cardiologist after surgery and don't be afraid to call and ask.

## Medicines

Your doctor will give you prescriptions before leaving the hospital. Take the medicine exactly as your doctor prescribes. I found that at first, if you make a time chart/list of the medications you need to take and when, it is very helpful. When you first arrive at home, you are still resting and or sleeping a lot, so a chart will help you stay on track with your medications. Do not take other medicines without telling or asking your doctors; they may want to approve or change those if they are not compatible with what they prescribed for you. With the chart you make, you can check it off as you take your medication, and let's face it, some of the medications are for pain or to help you sleep, so you may be fuzzy headed. Using your chart will really come in handy during that time. You could cause another problem with too much medication because you had forgotten you already took it, so the chart will keep you current and accurate

# Cardiac Surgery Discharge Concerns

You should seek immediate attention if you experience any of the following: Chest pains similar to pre-operative pain, shortness of breath not relieved by rest, chills or fever, sudden numbness or weakness in arms or legs, fainting spells, new onset of nausea, vomiting or diarrhea, bright red stool, heart rate faster than 150 beats/minute with shortness of breath or new irregular heart rate, coughing up bright red blood, sudden severe headache, or severe abdominal pain.

You should contact your local doctor if: You experience worsening ankle swelling or leg pain, sharp pain when taking in a deep breath, persistent bleeding or oozing from incisions, skin rash, acute gout flare-up, urinary tract infection, frequent urination, burning with urination, urgency to urinate, blood in your urine, weight gain more than one or two pounds in a day for two days, worsening shortness of breath, elevated temperature over a day's time, reddened wounds, warm to touch, swollen or any drainage, extreme fatigue, pain in calf that becomes worse when pointing toes towards the knee.

You may want to question the clinical nurse when: You are having concerns with postoperative recovery, discharge instructions, draining of wounds, questions related to surgery, management of symptoms, incision care, home health care, or directions for helpful community services or agencies in the area.

# CHAPTER 4

## Care of your Chest Incision

While still in the hospital, your doctor and nurses will take care of you and your incision. After you are discharged, most surgeons would agree that it is safe to wash your incision daily with mild soap and warm water. No vigorous scrubbing. Your nurse at discharge will tell you when it is okay to take a shower. The steri-strips usually fall off on their own. If after seven days after discharge, they have not, you may remove them. You may return home with stitches or staples in the incision in your leg. The doctor will remove these. You should try to avoid direct sunlight to your incisions; they will burn easily and cause discomfort. The scar may also pigment darker than the rest of the skin. Check with your doctor about application of lotions, creams, oils or powders. I always used creams that had vitamin E in them, and applied directly to the scar. I even took Vitamin E capsules and carefully sliced them open and applied the gel-like Vitamin E right on my scars. I found this practice worked very well for me.

Watch your incisions for increased tenderness, redness, swelling around the edges, or drainage. If you experience any of these conditions or fever, check with your doctor.

## Care Of Your Surgical Leg

If your doctor used a graft (artery for the bypass) from your leg, then try to avoid crossing your legs because this impairs circulation. Do not sit in one position or stand for a prolonged time. Elevating your leg on something when sitting will help with swelling. Check your leg daily for swelling. In time, you will not notice any difference from before the surgery.

## Elastic Stocking

The elastic stockings are sometimes prescribed by your doctor. Wear your elastic stocking while you are up and moving around for at least two weeks. The stockings will help decrease swelling, especially if you have a leg incision. You will not need to wear your stocking to bed, as your leg will be level.

## Going Home after Surgery

Five days after surgery, I was released from the hospital and sent home. Upon arriving back home, I wanted to make a visit to the middle school where I taught at that time. I entered the end of the building where I taught and went directly to my room. I said hello to the substitute and my students in that class and walked down the hall to the principal's office to visit as well. I spent about 30 minutes at the school and then went home to rest. Everyone at the school said that I looked good or great and of course I appreciated them lying, just to make me feel better. I had lost 22 pounds in 5 days and did not look good. But these were my friends and they were just saying something nice.

Frankly, I was scared with the thought and realization that I was home and away from the great nurses at the hospital. This feeling was taken over by my basic attitude to get up after you fall over a hurdle. I am, and was driven to push the envelope and get back to my life as I knew it. I had all my friends and family saying, take it easy, don't push too hard, be careful, maybe you shouldn't do that yet, and

I know they were all saying those things because they cared, but I had to do what I had to do. I had learned that there were treadmill tests that I would be taking to show progress. I asked the doctor about how that test would go, and then made that my first goal of achievement.

The test used would be the Bruce Protocol, which they described as seven 3-minute segments on the treadmill. You start off slow; on a flat tread, then after three minutes the speed is increased as well as the incline. Your level achieved in the test is measured in Mets, which could be a score of 1 to 18. If a patient scores 12 Mets, then everyone concerned is very happy. Of course, I didn't want a 12, I had to shoot for more and aim at the 18. In the test, everyone is different in terms of when they have to start running, instead of walking, when the speed and incline gets to that speed that you have to break into a jog. During the test, at the end of each 3-minute segment, the doctor or nurse comes upon your side and takes your blood pressure without you even stopping. This adds another margin of difficulty, as during that time, you cannot move your arm as you would naturally in a fast walk or jog. The jog soon turns into a run by the end of the test.

I fortunately, at that time owned a health club and in the club was a treadmill that had speed control and incline capabilities. Obviously, I did my training there so I could practice the 3-minute sections and then increase the speed and incline. I was monitoring my heart rate during my training, and I didn't know if there was a level that they wouldn't go past, but I did make the seven levels of the test at the health club only a few days before the scheduled test.

I was home for about five weeks from school and then returned to my teaching duty. In a staff meeting later that year, I thanked them for being so nice, saying I looked good when I returned, when I knew they were just being nice. I remember during that speech, I was very nervous and I thought my heart would beat right out of my chest. I can talk all day to my students and athletes, but in front of the whole staff is very tough for me. Likewise, I gave a speech of appreciation at my church, for all their prayers and letters of encouragement and for the Rev delivering me to the hospital and visiting me while in.

During the time at home right after surgery, I never felt more like an invalid. I was used to doing for myself and rush, rush, rushing all my life, so this was very humbling. The first time I felt handicapped was when I tried to open the pill bottles for my medication. Childproof? These things were too hard for me to squeeze and turn. These bottle were impermeable to me, I just couldn't open them. I had to have help getting them open and then I left them open, just in case no one was there when I needed them again. I had to sleep on the main floor, because my bed was upstairs and stairs were still too tough for me. That goal I accomplished in about two days, by using the railing for assistance. However, remember – if you start to climb the stairs and use the rail, it will flex your pectorals muscles and that needs to stay at a minimum.

Again I felt handicapped when I was grilling and the propane tank ran out. First of all, again, I couldn't squeeze hard enough to get the tank disconnected. Now you have to remember, I was into lifting weights and competing, and on a hand dynamometer, I had grip strength of just less than 180 pounds with my right and 160 pounds with my left, and now I couldn't open a pill bottle or use vise grips to loosen the propane tank. I was feeling real dependent. When I traveled in the car, just riding, I had to have a pillow by my chest for protection, in case of a little bump or accident. While I wanted to be independent and not have people wait on me, I needed them. My Mom stayed with me for a couple weeks after surgery to help out. She was a Godsend and still is.

Three days after I arrived home, I ignored the Doc's orders and went to the weight room and started doing seated dumbbell curls with five pounds in each hand. I remember the Doc saying that a gallon of milk was too much, and I had that figured at eight pounds, so I convinced myself that I was safe to do reps with the five-pound dumbbells. Now when I say I went to the weight room, It wasn't that far away. We had built a 21' x 26' room on the side of the house that was better equipped than most health Spas or weight rooms. By then, I was in the process of selling one health club to our south and still owned the club to the north. I started my walks outside in our small town and most people in town knew what I had gone through. Like many small towns, people knew and cared what was going on with one of theirs. Many odd jobs around the house had been taken care of by people anonymously and no one even admitted that they took part. It was very much appreciated. Many brought over prepared meals, cookies and goodies for a number of weeks.

I started my walks around the block and then again, kept increasing the distance and number of times per day. I also mixed in protein powder with low fat milk and other ingredients like bananas, strawberries, wheat germ, and flavors like chocolate to make protein shakes, that I took daily, and even two and three times per day. I really wanted to return to power lifting competition, so I made that as one of my goals. Surgery was in October, so when I returned home in Michigan, the weather was good enough to walk outside. I had follow-up visits with the surgeon for a couple weeks and all was progressing very quickly. I soon was released from his care.

# 1<sup>st</sup> Treadmill Test

This test would determine how I was doing, and if I could return to my job as a teacher. It was important to me to do well as I mentioned earlier. I had set the date of this test like a power lifting meet date, where I got myself ready for competition. It was me against the treadmill and my goal was to last as long as possible into the test before the doctor would shut it down. I arrived at the hospital, where the test would take place and took my sweat pants and sweatshirt off, so I was down to my running shorts and tank top. I started to stretch and warm up with some trunk twists.

The nurses were in and out for the next 10-15 minutes and remarked how they had been doing these tests on people for a long time, and this was the first time someone was warming up for it. I said I wouldn't be happy with just passing the test, I wanted to blow the lid off of it, and so I needed to warm up. I asked my cardiologist when he entered, what was the record of Mets from this test. He answered that one guy, who was trying to qualify to be an Air Force pilot had completed the test in all of 21 minutes. I said had he had heart surgery, and he answered: Heavens no and he was in his mid-twenties. He continued to say that 12 was the highest Mets of a heart patient. I knew I would be over 12 and wanted to go for the pilot's record. I told the doctor of my intention and he said: Well, we can leave you on the test until you reach 100% working heart rate, meaning during the test when your heart beats faster and faster as the test gets tougher, you will reach a point when you will be at the max of your heart being 100% filled by the bypasses and it will beat. If you go beyond that point and your heart rate goes up again and beats before it is 100% full of blood, it will appear to the test results that you have a blockage, when actually, you have just put forth an effort greater than 100% working heart rate. We will have to shut off the treadmill and slowly bring you into your cool down with lesser speed and incline. You may be ready to go on, but we cannot let you do that.

## Test Time

We started the test, and the first phase was so slow, it was almost annoying, but it was part of the test. I progressed through the levels and they took my blood pressure each time. I was also completely wired for an EKG (Electro Cardiogram). The box had to be hooked to my shorts, which I didn't plan for, and the waistband of my shorts was not that tight, so the heavy box sort of tugged on that side of my shorts. If I had planned ahead for that box, I would have brought a belt, so the box could be hooked to it.

In the sixth level with only one more level, I had one minute to go, when the doctor said, "You have already passed all expectations that we wanted to see. You are well over 12 Mets and your heart rate is getting close to when we will have to stop you." I said, "Let me go as long as you can." Frankly, I had just started to sweat. I was breathing hard, had already broken into a run, and knew as soon as they increased the speed and incline, that my heart would jump again. With all of my past cross country training, decathlon and road races, I tried to summon all the control I had. I took a couple of cleansing breaths and tried to calm myself and I actually lowered my heart rate a little. Shortly after we increased to the seventh and last level, my heart rate jumped as expected and almost a minute into the last three minutes, the doctor gave the signal to the nurse to begin the slow-down. I ended the test with a score of 16 Mets. I was disappointed, but also knew that he couldn't let me go any more without risking his own beliefs and training. They said we would repeat this test in six months, to make sure everything was going well. Now I know that you are way ahead of me already and yes, you got it. He just gave me a new target date and test to make all 21 minutes six months from then, and surpass the mark I had just set.

# CHAPTER 5

## Post-operative Activity

S top any activity that causes shortness of breath, feeling faint, chest pain, or irregular heart rate. Rest until recovered. If recovery takes longer than 20 minutes, notify your doctor.

SHOWERS:
It is okay to resume showers when your doctor approves; avoid extremely hot water, soaking in baths, and make sure you are not experiencing any dizziness.

DRESS:
You will want to wear comfortable, loose-fitting clothes that do not put pressure on your incisions. Sweat pants if you have a leg incision, and shirts that are not tight. Avoid clothing that would rub on your incisions.

REST:
You should balance your rest with your recovery activities. Plan your walks, followed by a 20-30 minute rest. Schedule a rest after eating as well.

WALKING:

This is your primary activity for a few weeks. Your walking will increase circulation throughout the body and the heart muscle. You should plan to increase your activity of walking by distance or time, whichever is easier for you to figure. Walk at your own pace, but pace is another variable that you can use when you are recovering. Make sure you stop and rest when you need to. This is not a race; you are on the road to recovery, so listen to your body.

Everyone progresses at a different rate after surgery, depending on many variables such as age, weight, and other painful joints to name a few. Pace yourself, don't plan a bunch of activities back-to-back. You must schedule in your rest periods. When it is too cold or too hot to walk outside, then try to get to a mall or even walk at your local school in the evenings. If it is below 40 or above 80 degrees, think about an indoor alternative place to walk. During recovery, as you build your strength and tolerance up, you will be able to handle cold and heat better.

STAIRS:
Make sure this activity is approved by your doctor. When climbing stairs, take them at a slow pace, watch for dizziness, stop and rest when you're tired. When using the rail, use it for balance only, do not pull yourself up with your arms. Let your legs do the work. Pulling on the rail will flex your chest muscles and possibly cause a problem.

SEXUAL:
For many people, it is about two to four weeks after discharge, unless instructed differently by your doctor. You can resume sexual relations when you feel comfortable. If you can climb a flight of stairs without using the railing and not be short of breath, then you are probably ready, but it is still a good idea to ask your nurse or doctor for more detailed information.

DRIVING:
Riding as a passenger is fine anytime. You should avoid getting behind the wheel yourself, or bicycling or motorcycle riding for six weeks after surgery. Your sternum, or breastbone, needs to

heal. Your reactions and movements are limited and lower at this time. When traveling, you should get out and walk every two hours.

LIFTING:
Usually, you should wait six weeks before lifting anything more than a gallon of milk, which is 8.2 pounds. You should not put too much strain on your sternum while it is healing. This includes pushing, pulling and lifting movements, including things like carrying children, groceries, suitcases, mowing the grass, vacuuming, moving furniture, and shoveling. Avoid holding your breath during any activity; this includes while lifting anything or when using the rest room.

WORK:
It will be up to your surgeon when you can return to work, but most patients will begin to feel like returning to light work about six to twelve weeks after surgery. This of course depends on the type of work that you do. If you work in a non-physical position, you may return more quickly than someone in a physically demanding job. You may also look at your situation as, when do I *have* to go back? Again, your doctor can help with this by putting in writing that you are or are not ready to return to work. Some employers will require a letter of release for work from your doctor before allowing you back to work. My position was unique; I wanted to push the envelope and get back to work ASAP. If I was in construction work, I might not have been so cocky. Just make sure that when you return to work, it is safe for you and all those around you.

## Rehabilitation

What is Cardiac Rehabilitation? Cardiac Rehabilitation is what people do after having bypass, valve replacement, transplant, pacemaker, or other cardiac surgical procedures to get going again. Your support group is made up of your doctor(s) nurses, exercise physiologists, and nutritionist to help you feel well again.

FIRST:
Early after surgery, while still in the hospital, you will start your light walking and possibly stairs.

SECOND:
As an early outpatient of cardiac rehabilitation, you will work to improve endurance and learn to deal with your reduced capacity to do the things you were used to.

THIRD:
You will work towards an ongoing exercise program, set and strive for goals such as independent life style and returning to work, and get educated in prevention training for future heart trouble.

FINALLY:
You are practicing a wellness program with improved diet ("heart smart" eating) and lifestyle changes including exercising three to four times per week and stopping any habits detrimental to your health, such as smoking.

## When To Resume Usual Activities

In the first six weeks you may participate in the following activities: Light housekeeping like dusting, setting the table, washing dishes, folding clothes. For outdoor activities, chores such as potting plants and trimming flowers, attending sports events, and walking. You may also read, do needlework, cook, climb stairs, shop, go to restaurants, church, and movies, use a treadmill or stationary bike, play cards, shampoo hair and some small mechanical jobs. Until six weeks have passed after surgery, keep in mind that activities have an eight to ten pound limit or less. Remember, your first week of the six weeks will be in the hospital.

After 6 weeks, you may be able to return to work, if your job does not require lifting and the return is approved by your doctor. You can now add heavy housework, such as vacuuming, sweeping, laundry, ironing, light aerobics, and walking the dog, if the dog is light on the leash. You may also start mowing the lawn, if it is not a strenuous push mower, raking leaves, traveling, and fishing.

After 3 months, you should be able to return to most jobs, even if they include lifting. Once again, check with your doctor. Other activities that should feel fine at this point are shoveling snow, scrubbing floors, digging. You can probably return to most sports activities such as tennis, bowling, hunting, jogging, bicycling, golfing, weight lifting, swimming, water skiing, skydiving, softball, baseball, and soccer. Yes, I said skydiving.

## Exercise Guidelines

When you return to any exercise, stop that exercise if you experience shortness of breath, dizziness, leg cramping, unusual fatigue or chest pain. Once again: Listen to your body. If it says whoa, then whoa. If it says go, then go. When you do exercise; be aware of your pulse. Check your pulse by counting the heartbeats for 15 seconds and multiplying by four. That is your heart rate per minute. If you have a resting heart rate of 70, then your working heart rate is upwards of 140, but again, listen to your body and check with your physician with any exercise program you are considering. In time, your doctor will give you a clean bill of health or describe the restrictions to you, and then listen to him.

## Getting BackTo Normal Activities

This is not recommended, or even normal, but I actually went back to performing the bench press exercise within four weeks after surgery. I was very careful when I brought the bar down to my chest, because my sternum was still held together with wires. I continued to work on my bench press and on being a competitive power lifter as I was before surgery. I wanted to get back at it ASAP. My pectorals muscles responded right away and built back up to where they were in just a few weeks. By doing so, this caused a stretch on the scar that was left up the middle of my chest, over the sternum. Keloid tissue then formed within the scar and it got thicker and thicker and hard. It was soon nearly the size of a pencil, so I then had to pursue how to get rid of that. I went to a dermatologist and he started cortisone shots into the scar from top to bottom about every half-inch apart. They stung like bee stings, but then I would rub the area and the scar tissue started to break up. With each subsequent visit to the dermatologist, the space between shots increased to 1" apart, then 1-½" apart and so on, for about 7 visits and then the scar was back to flat. This process took a number of weeks and as I said, stung a lot, but it was worth it when the scar was flat again.

I also added to my workouts the full gamut of lifts for power lifting with the squat and dead lift and auxiliary lifts that help to increase these lifts. By this time, I had added a goal of getting back on the competitive platform for power lifting in the sub-masters division, which is for lifters over the age of 35. So I added that goal to the two ideas I had discussed in the hospital of jumping out of a plane and playing basketball with my brother again.

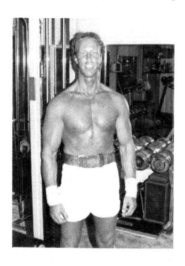

I went back to teaching within five weeks after surgery and added going to our health club after school to continue my road back to competition. It was that following summer, eight months after surgery that I returned to the competitive platform in power lifting. As I mentioned before, I was in a separation/attempt to reconcile, and separated again, with an eventual divorce in the summer of 1990. In the divorce, the health clubs did not stay in my pocession and life changed dramatically again. This was a time when my optimism was truly tested. There were times that trying to see the glass as half-full was very difficult. Many times, after heart surgery, the patient will go through depression when they figure out what things they can no longer do. At this point, I found that considering the alternative, of not making it through the surgery, helped to push the depression thoughts out of my mind. But then add a divorce shortly after it; the depression was hard to fight. It was then that I had to dig deep for my core values of survival and always striving to look for the good in any situation.

The following school year, I returned to coaching at the school, as my health clubs were gone and I didn't have a facility to continue coaching power lifting. Coaching has been such a huge part of my life that I returned to coaching at the high school. There is more about the return to coaching later.

## Starting Some New Activities

*"We don't stop playing because we grow old; We grow old because we stop playing."*

*-George Bernard Shaw*

## It's 3-On-3 Macker Time

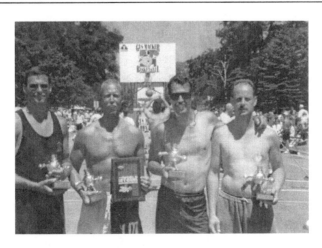

When school got out in June of 1990, and I had set up plans with my brother to enter some Macker 3-on-3 basketball tournaments. He would hook up with a teammate from his town and I with one in my town, so we could practice one-on-one with our local teammates. I found a student athlete's Dad to team up with to play in the Mackers, and he started lifting weights with me as well. We became lifting partners and good friends as well as teammates on the basketball court. He had previously played basketball for CMU, so I picked a good teammate; he was 6'4" to my 6'2" and he still had game. We worked out three to six days per week, both in the weight room and on the basketball court. I could out-muscle him a little and he had a better shot. We pushed hard on each other in training, as that was the style of play in these 3-on-3 tournaments; it could get quite rough at times. In these contests, when you are on offense and try to score, the defense will hack you on purpose, because it's up to the offensive player to call the foul and chances are, you will miss the shot and that would be mission accomplished by the defense. It's part of the game, so you plan for it.

We then entered the Belding Macker and started our playing together. It was great playing with my brother again. In all reality, my brother is the much better player. When he was a senior and I was a junior on our varsity basketball team, I usually got in only if he fouled out. That was a difficult position for me, to root for my brother, while hoping to get in, which meant he would have to foul out. What a struggle, eh? He also made CMU's basketball team as my partner did, and played one year for CMU as well.

Our Mackers added the Ludington competition as well. In one of our years in Belding, we were lucky enough to win the tournament, and we did it in the worst-case scenario possible. We lost the first game on Friday night, and then had to come back through the entire losers bracket with four games on Saturday and seven games on Sunday, including having to win twice in the finals, as it was a double elimination tournament. We also won the sportsmanship award at times in other Mackers we played in around the state as well. We continued our Macker involvement for a number of years, until we realized that it was time to put up our shoes, but it wasn't due to any heart problems. I really enjoyed those times playing with my brother again and my local partner will be a friend in my heart forever.

## Jumping Out Of An Air Plane

It finally happened in the summer 1994, my local Macker partner and I discussed the desire to sky dive. When I learned that he was interested too, we started looking for the opportunity to do just that. He found an advertisement about a class and a jump and we signed up. We took the class together, which was a one-day, several hour

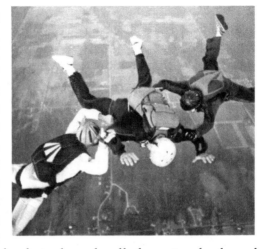

class. We learned how to land, tuck and roll, how to check and untangle the lines to our chutes, and exactly what was going to happen during the jump. There was class, videos and jumping off of rungs of a ladder to simulate the landing. We were told to wait for a call when they had time to arrange for the pilot and plane in our local town. Upon arrival for the class, which took about four hours, we had to fill out many forms. I'm afraid that I had to lie when filling it out, or the jump would not have taken place and they would have rejected me. Samples: Do you have a bad heart? NO. Do you have a bad back? NO. Do you have bad knees? NO. Is there any other reason you should not jump out of a plane? NO. Now, please don't try this at home. I do not recommend fudging the answers on any forms, but at that point in my life, I was blinded by the need to jump out of an airplane. It was only about 10 days later; we got the call, and learned we would be making our jump that weekend. My friend and I arrived with some of our kids to watch and we prepared for the jump. We could only go up one at a time in the small Cessna plane. We did "rock-paper-scissors" and my partner won, so I watched as he did his jump with total excitement. In the plane were the two instructors, a photographer and the student. My friend had scraped the knuckles of his hand in his landing and they were bleeding, but he never knew it due to the adrenalin rush he had going.

My excitement in waiting for my partner to take his jump was out of control. I was like a kid in a candy store who couldn't touch anything. He jumped, landed, and couldn't stop raving about how incredible it was. Next, the instructors repacked their chutes and up we went and it was my turn. The small plane went up and up and it was like the anticipation of riding a roller coaster where you are slowly pulled up and finally break over the top.

We did get lucky enough to have a professional sky diving photographer on hand, as our instructors knew him and he was in town, up from Florida visiting his hometown in that area in Michigan. This was a huge bonus for us, even though it added some more cost to the experience We were going to have a video and 36 still shots from his 35-millimeter camera. Both cameras were mounted into his helmet and a cord went down the inside of his sleeve to his hand, to control the shutter of the still camera and the video camera.

Our climb up finally reached two miles, or 10,560 feet. The pilot started his slow down approach to the jump site, so that I would be exiting the plane at the right spot, so I would end up hitting the airport runway below. About that time, they threw the side door open, which swung upward, and the wind sound was very loud. It was then that the realization really hit. When I looked out, all I could focus on was the mile square sections below me and sections of trees, (), and had to search for the airport. All of us would be jumping, except the pilot of course, and my instructor told me that no one rides down; the only way down is out the door. The plane slowed down to around 60mph, then the photographer exited first, but he didn't jump. He held onto the framework of the wing and went out very near the end of the wing, but I wasn't watching him. I was too nervous to know where he was.

Next, one instructor went out followed quickly by me and then the other instructor. All three of us were balanced on a small flat platform above the wheel of the plane and hanging onto the angled crossbar supporting the wing. We were all under the wing, feeling the 60 mph wind, and as instructed, I gave the count and we all bailed, let loose of the wing, at once. My jump suit had loop handles by my hips and outside my shoulders, and the instructors held onto me there. We were not tandem, strapped together; we all had our own chutes. Upon starting our free fall, we were heading straight down, head first, and I was spellbound momentarily and just watching and taking in everything I could see. Within 10 seconds, we were at a speed of 120mph and my instructors using hand signals reminded me to arch, so I did.

We stayed in the free fall until we had descended to 5,000 feet on my altimeter, or about 1 mile. The instructor again reminded me with a hand signal it was time to pull the ripcord for the chute to deploy. As soon as the student does pull the cord, then the instructors let go and free fall some more on their own. The photographer, who had wing-like pieces of cloth under his arms in his jump suit, was flying around me the entire time and snapping pictures and filming. He was nearly close enough in front of me to touch at one point, so I waved to him, and that you can clearly see on my video. He also descended faster, landed and continued with the video from the ground and followed me in my landing. So I ended up with a complete flight video from him, and was given the roll of 35mm shots to develop. It was a great bonus, and how I had access to the pictures you see.

The student's chute is a truck, as they called it, meaning a very big canopy, giving a slow ride down, and softer landing. What I learned in class was to check the deployment of my chute, in case anything was tangled, how to untangle it and if that didn't work, how to release it and deploy your backup shute, and then check that one. If that one didn't work, I think you would be down on the ground by then anyway. Upon the landing, we learned to pull the toggles to slow down before contacting the ground, and then drop and do a forward roll to avoid jarring the knees of a beginner. I made the simple roll in the grass next to the airport runway, came right back up and started gathering up the lines of the chute. This was another instruction from class, teaching if there as a wind and it catches your chute, it can drag you along the ground pretty quickly, so we were taught to gather and wrap up our chutes immediately. Other than the birth of my three children, this was the single biggest adrenalin rush that I had to date. To be flying, out of control, with reckless abandonment at 120 mph, and solely reliant on a ripcord opening the chute to land. "WHAT A RUSH!" Just like my partner, after landing, I couldn't take the smile off my face and couldn't stop talking about every aspect of the entire experience. It was amazing.

I have been asked if I would do it again. I probably would not, for two reasons: 1.) Like my marathon run, now I can say "I did that," and 2.) the total cost with the class, jump and film was near $400 and I can think of better things to do with $400. Things I haven't done yet, or, better yet, bills to pay.

## Returning To Power Lifting

Eight months after surgery, I returned to the lifting platform, ready to compete again. The Sub-Masters State finals, which were for the lifter between 35 years and 40, were taking place in Grand Rapids. I competed in the 198-pound class after some hard training and was victorious that day with a squat of 500 pounds, bench of 350 pounds, and dead lift of 540 pounds for a 1390 pounds. I received some great awards that day, which I still have. I felt good about making the comeback. I was also a host of many power lifting meets and continued doing so after surgery. It was shortly after that, when I was inducted into the Administrative portion of the Michigan Power Lifting Hall of Fame. This was also the time that my divorce was final and the result of that was me being totally out of the health club business. Without the facility to train, I returned to training at the school that I taught at and then returned to coaching at the school, soon after that. I had to stay busy, and the coaching definitely did that for me.

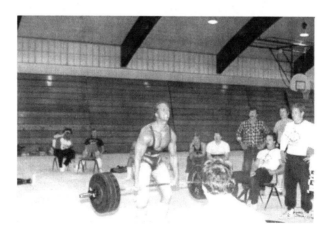

## Return To Coaching At School

The first sport that I returned to was varsity volleyball. I had coached varsity volleyball for five seasons back in 1978-1982, and we actually upped the school record of wins in a season four out of those five seasons. In 1983, I opened health clubs and was too busy to continue coaching at the school, but now my health clubs were gone. So I returned to volleyball when there was a vacancy in the varsity position in the 1990-1991 season. In Michigan, volleyball has been a winter sport for a long time, while most states compete in volleyball in the fall. Litigation to change the season in Michigan to the Fall took many years and the switch was made for the fall season of 2007, so Michigan is now in line with the rest of the country. When I returned, it was a tough year for the team, as I inherited a team that had trained no one for the most important spot, the setter, and there were only one or two players who could touch the top of the net. I knew we had our work cut out for us. The team worked very hard on serving the heck out of the ball and became great passers.

We only won 11 matches that year, but gained a lot of respect for being able to cover the floor. We made it difficult for our opponents to find the floor on our side; we just kept digging it back up. That type of team can only last so long against attacking teams, but we made them earn it, losing a lot of games by just a few points. That was our 1990-91 season and it was great being back in the VB coaching chair, and I set my sights on building a team to be reckoned with. Our record that first year back was 11-26-3, so I needed to step up and re-build the program. I worked hard to turn that around from the 7$^{th}$ grade on up to varsity. The next year in 1992, we were over 500 with a 16-14-10 record followed by six straight years of breaking the school record wins in a season. The old record was 27 wins in a season and we improved that to 38 in 1993 and continued to move that record up to the existing record of 56 wins in 1998, which is still the mark to beat after the 2008 season.

It was in November of 2002 when I had my second open heart

43

surgery, and the school assigned an interim coach with team until my return I could return. The team accumulated 41 wins in that, my final season, 29 of which were after my return to the team. We had set a goal of 50 for that team before the season started, and I feel they would have achieved it, had I been with them from the beginning of the season. During that season, the team accomplished a win late in the season that gave me my 500th win. By the end of the season, I retired from volleyball with 516 varsity wins, in 18 seasons, all of which I credit to the kids' hard work. When we hit number 500, the parents of the team had rallied and had a celebration planned that started right after the match. It was both humbling and exciting.

The next sport I returned to was track and field, also in 1991. As I mentioned earlier, I started running track in elementary school and through middle and high school and I ran the decathlon in college. I was ready to get back into coaching both because I loved it and because I needed to stay busy. I've always been a workaholic and staying busy after the divorce was important for me. Once I started coaching track again , it all came back to me quickly. We were very successful in the next decade. We amassed a record of 110 wins to only one loss in dual meets in the next 10 years. We had one of the best-undefeated records going in the state when we lost number 70 by just one point. We were State Champions in 1994 plus many Regional and League championships during that time frame. My last season was the spring of 2002, giving me 18 years in that sport as well. It was always a great pleasure and very fulfilling.

The next Sport I returned to was cross country in 1993. I first started coaching CC as soon as I came to that school in 1975. I coached for six years and I started Girls Cross Country at our school. Now, I was back at the helm, running the program. That year, we had only seven athletes, but they all had hearts of lions and they managed to do the impossible by winning the State Championship meet and were crowned number one in the State. It was such a fantastic and memorable time for all seven of those athletes and the school and the community. There were five cameras per athlete taking pictures of every one of the athletes and newspaper interviews and medals for all the athletes, team trophy and more. This feat, also earned me "Coach of the Year." Over the years, I was given that award two more times, which was a great honor.

During meets, when my kids were competing, I was not an idle coach. I could be seen running zigzag patterns all over the course when my team was running. My last season in 2001, I chased my team furiously all season long and only three weeks before my second open heart surgery. Obviously I chased the runners without any knowledge of the aneurysm that was in my chest, which was like a time bomb. That is what the doctors told me at the time of my heart catheterization when they found it. They said one part was actually leaking blood. I'm glad it didn't explode during those competition days for a number of reasons, and mostly for the simple fact that it would be terrible for a team to lose their coach that way at a meet.

# CHAPTER 6

## Diet

Your doctor will probably recommend that you follow a low fat, no salt added diet after you are discharged. It is a good idea to have less than 30% of your calories from fat. Eat less saturated fat and cholesterol, and control your weight. The American Heart Association recommends that saturated fatty acid intake should be 8–10% of your calories. Polyunsaturated fatty acid intake should be up to 10% of your calories. Monounsaturated fatty acids make up the rest of the total fat intake, about 10-15% of total calories. Cholesterol intake should be less than 300 milligrams per day. Sodium intake should be no more than 2,400 milligrams (2.4 grams) per day.

Avoid adding salt to cooking or at the table. Begin making changes to your diet when your appetite returns after returning home. I have always gone by the idea of, "If it swims or flies, you can eat it, as long as you don't fry it." Eat plenty of fruits and vegetables, stay away from fried foods and red meat. It's usually what you put on your food that is not so good for you, such as the butter, the salt, the dressing, and so on. Get the idea? I heard that the average American eats around 150 pounds of sugar and fats per year. To counter balance all that sugar that turns to fat, there are some foods that can help. Artichokes are great to regulate sugars and actually help to raise your HDL's, the good cholesterol, and help to lower the bad cholesterol, LDL. Another one that lowers your LDL is squash; you can remember this by saying squash will help squash your LDL. Onions and onion juice will help to raise your HDL's. Persimmons lowers your LDL's. Preservatives and additives in foods that add to the shelf-life of these foods and products do the opposite for us. If you want to preserve and add to your life, don't eat products that have preservatives and additives in them. Garlic has always been a "heart smart" food as well.

It is important that you check with your doctor or a nutritionist before establishing your diet for yourself, because they are licensed to do so where I am not.

If weight is an issue for you, and you are now keeping a closer watch, then weigh in consistently. Weigh in at the same time each morning after you urinate and before you eat breakfast, and use the same scales in the same position on the floor, wearing virtually the same clothes, or always nude. This will be a consistent reading. It will be the least that you will weigh all day, as you have just slept and haven't eaten for about eight to 12 hours. Keep track of your weight, and it may help for you to keep track of your eating at first, as it keeps you on track.

Make sure that if you gain two pounds or more over night, contact your doctor right away. Seldom, but enough to keep track, if you gain weight over night, the doctor may want to check if you are building up fluids from weeping inside your chest cavity.

## Smoking

Please don't get me wrong; I am not condemning anyone who smokes. I realize full well the addictive quality of nicotine found in cigarettes, and people do have the freedom of choice. It has never been my choose to smoke.

There are numerous studies out there that have proven that smoking is not advantageous to your health and heart. If you already have a tendency for heart trouble, then why make it even worse. We all know that in baseball, you get three strikes. Poor genetics for heart disease is strike one, take up smoking, strike two, but I wasn't given a choice for my strike one, and someone who smokes does. It is my understanding that when a person first starts smoking, their blood pressure will elevate. It may level off and come back down, but for the most part, smoking causes a slight increase in your BP. Besides the obvious risk of cancer and increased heart problems, it is hard for me to understand why a person would smoke. I have spent all my life knowing that my life would be shorter than the average American and have worked out to stay in shape to help prolong it. I try to eat right to help, and still had two bypass surgeries before I was 50.

A smoker has to have heard that you take seven minutes off your life with every cigarette, plus the time you wasted in smoking it. I have a hard time understanding when I practice the things to help me live longer and people who smoke are doing something that can cause death to come earlier. And yes, I do have family members who smoke, but I don't hound them about it. It's their life and they choose what they want to do; I'm coming at it with a different view, my view.

# CHAPTER 7

## Second Surgery

I t was the fall of 2002 and my knee was bothering me more and
more, so I returned to my local orthopedic surgeon in northern
Michigan. I was determined that it was time to re-enter and fix some
meniscus problems and do some basic clean up of the scar tissue. On
November 4th my knee surgery took place. A few days later, I
developed a rash around my knee that was the same shape and length
of the wrap-around ice pack used on my knee for swelling. I was
prescribed a seven-day steroid pack to help with this problem. I had
some reservations about taking anything that had steroids in it with
my heart history, but I trusted my doctor. Just the second day into the
steroid pack, I started to have chest pains, mild at first and then
harder. This concerned me, but I stayed on the medication schedule. I
had a lot going on in my life, and I needed to get the knee problems
behind me. I had just finished coaching varsity girls' cross country
and my varsity volleyball season was about to begin. I had planned
the knee surgery for the short break that was between my cross-
country season and the volleyball season.

I went with my good friend, Sir, to the MIVCA (Michigan
Volleyball Coaches Association) clinic in Battle Creek for the
weekend. Sir and I attended this event annually. I brought my
crutches, but was on my second day of attempting to walk without

them. I carried my portable chair and shoulder bag to the clinic events and made my way around the booths and bought things for my team for the upcoming season. Friday evening after feeling bushed from the day's events, I retired early to the hotel room, while Sir attended a volleyball match in Grand Rapids. I was propped up in the bed watching TV by 9:00 p.m. and slowly got thick eyed. Then I had it. The chest pain was back in full force, like I had felt back in 1989. I lay down on my side and tried to relax and put into use the breathing techniques I learned way back in birthing class. The pain continued and I considered my options: Try to get a hold of Sir, but, no he was out of town. Call my wife; but no, that would worry her too much. Call the hotel front desk, but, no, they would call 911 and all heck would break loose and the hype and excitement might all be for a false alarm. So I thought I would just ride it out. Then I thought I should at least get up and write a note to my wife and kids and say how much I loved them just in case this wasn't a false alarm. I finally, through my relaxation exercises, felt the pains start to subside and I fell off to sleep as I was considering these options. I may point out at this point that I am narcoleptic. I can fall asleep within about three breaths after hitting a comfortable position, and I have used it many times to escape stress and/or pain.

The next day, I took it real slow and attended the clinic sessions and Sir and I headed home. On Sunday, at home, I didn't do anything physical and had no chest pains. I hoped the pains were only from the medications and I was done with them, so maybe the pains would be done too. On Monday I went to school by 6:45 a.m. and went to the weight room and got in a workout before school started, as I always did. My first hour class reported to the weight room by 8:10, and by 8:15 my chest started to hurt again. Within the next half hour, I arranged on the phone for the school secretary to find me a substitute, as I could tell that I needed to go home. At the conclusion of first hour, I walked across campus to the school nurse to have her take my blood pressure. It was good at 125/80, so I continued out to my second hour class in the art room. There I made a couple more calls to find a sub quickly, as the pain was unrelenting. They did find someone to cover for me and I packed my things and drove home, which was only a half mile from the school.

Once home, I lay down on the couch and tried to rest and then called my wife at work to let her know what was going on. She called back moments later and said she was coming home so we could go to the doctor or hospital. She arrived home and we went to the emergency room at the hospital and they ran many tests. All the tests said that everything was fine with the heart, but I knew better. The EKG read normal, everything read normal and they said it was indigestion, but I knew better. Part of the reason I went to the hospital was that my cardiologist was at the hospital doing a treadmill test on another patient and I wanted to see him. I asked the emergency room personnel to talk to him and tell him that I wanted to see him. They contacted him, and sent a message back that he had seen the test results and things seemed OK, and to make an appointment with his office.

When we arrived back home, I called my cardiologist's office to make the appointment and got in to see him the next day. That visit proved to be much of the same, with all tests showing everything was normal, but again I knew better. I started to have chest pains while in his office and they ran another EKG, which again was normal. I spoke frankly with my doctor and said, "All these tests are missing something. I know my body and what it's telling me. I knew for my first five-way bypass 13 years ago and I know now and I want a heart catheterization and I would like one ASAP." Doc knew I was serious and knew that I had been right-on before and thankfully took the ball and got it scheduled. We walked out to the secretary together as she called Saginaw and Lansing. I had said I would take the one who had the first opening, as I knew time was a factor for me. Lansing was able to get me in the next morning, and we were on our way to finding out exactly what was going on.

So then it was off to Lansing for my wife and me to Ingham Hospital that same day. The next morning I was ready for the heart cath. I was mentally prepared for having surgery, because I know my system and I can feel changes and problems. It had been 13 years since my first bypass surgery and the surgeon had said that the bypasses were good for 10 to 12 years. I wasn't sure if that meant that they would clog again or a vein used from the leg has a longevity rating of 10 to 12 years before they don't work any more. No matter which one, I knew I was ready again.

With the recent developments of the stent, I was really planning on a quick in and out, pop a few stents in there and it would be back to work for me. After all, volleyball season was starting and I had work to do. I have always been an athlete and coached athletics and believe you have to psych up for upcoming challenges and events. I was psyched to have some stents put in, and then win 50 matches that season in volleyball.

Well it was heart catherization time, so I was prepared for the procedure and in we went. There was a doctor and a couple of nurses on hand. I was lying on the table and they prepared to insert the catheter into my groin. We were all talking during the procedure and the doctor remarked how this one was pretty routine. The staff was saying, look what good shape this guy is in, low body fat; this is going to be an easy one. I remember there was a radio playing quietly in the background, set to an oldies channel, which was good for my taste. The doctor was singing along with the radio and a nurse said to him, "You can't sing during these." And he said: "Sure we can, this is a routine one." Then I said, "Leave him alone, this is a good song." Then I heard, "Click," and the radio was off and someone said: "Holly crap, what is that?"

I said, "Hey guys, good song, routine, what's up?" The doctor said. "We'll be right with you Mr. Burke." in a noticeable change to professional talk, and no more fun. Then there was quieter talking. I heard, "Have you ever seen anything like that before?" and the answer, "No." Then another doctor was invited in to look at the aneurysm they had found and again the question: "Have you ever seen anything like that?" The second doctor said "Sure, every day." Then after a pause, he said. "No, I never have, not in 20 years of this." The Doctor, who was on a rolling chair, rolled up towards my head. He said: "We've found an aneurysm and I'm afraid we're going to have to go in." I did not know what an aneurysm was, so I said: "Go in, meaning to put in stents?" He replied: "No, I mean we're going to have to crack you open again." I paused as that news took a second to sink in and then I said: "Oh, well you're going to have to give me a little time for that, I am going to have to psych up for open heart, I was prepared mentally for some stents, not to be cracked open again." The Doctor said: "I understand, but don't plan on going home."

At this time, both doctors and one nurse left the room and one nurse stayed with me. I could see the doctors through a glass wall informing my wife, Rhonda, about the aneurysm and the fact that there was going to be an open heart surgery scheduled. I saw her head drop and she brought her hands up over her face and was starting to cry. The nurse "angel" that stayed with me was sitting on the rolling chair up by my head and we were talking quietly. I asked her how many doctors performed the open heart surgeries here at Ingham. She replied that there were eight cardiac surgeons. I then asked if she had kids, to which she replied yes. Then I asked which doctor would she ask to do the surgery on her child. She said that she would have Doctor ---, and she named him. She also said, it would be best if I didn't mention that she gave me the name of the doctor to use. I said "Of course," I then asked her to go tell the doctors still talking to my wife that I would like that particular doctor to perform the surgery. One of the doctors came back into the room and said. "Do you know Doctor so-and-so?" And I said, "No, I just want the best to do the surgery." He said, "OK, you've got him." I never had a chance to thank that angel who was one of my nurses.

I was then admitted to the hospital and awaited word. Rhonda and I and my kids spent the evening talking. My parents, brothers and other family members were all called and they all came to visit before the surgery. Crandall, my oldest daughter, my first born will always be my first baby, was there right away and helped me by picking up materials from school that I could work on and get things ready for me being gone from my teaching/coaching jobs. She is a great organizer and planner, a trait I passed on to her.

My other daughter, who was on a basketball scholarship at Colgate University in New York, somehow, through the NCAA arranged to fly home to see me before surgery. We are a family of athletes and her season was just starting and this would make her miss her first game, which I didn't want to happen, for her and her team, as she was the captain, and an integral part of the program. But the loving daughter that she is would not have been able to perform in the game, with her Daddio on a slab, and the coaches knew that, so there she was, with me. I don't even know whom to thank and my appreciation goes out to everyone who helped in this possibility that I could see my baby and get hugs and kisses and more bonding before surgery. I told her all would be fine, and she should try to refocus on her game as soon as she could after surgery and for her to play for me. That was hard to say, because I loved watching her play and it choked me up to say: "Play for me." My adopted daughter, Erin, was also there. Her father died before she was born and I have been the only father that she has known. She was also very moved with my condition and it was wonderful to have her there with me and to be with her mother, Rhonda, who had lost her previous husband, Erin's father 22 years before. Erik, my son, was in his junior year of high school basketball season at Traverse City Central High School, and it bothered me again that he was missing practice and possibly a game, because we are all about athletics. I am so proud of the man he has become. I told him not to worry, that: "I'll be back," in my best Arnold impersonation. And I would be there to watch many more of his football and basketball games, and track meets. Without any fear of his masculinity, we kissed and he told me he loved me and I him.

My Mother and Step-Dad, whom I call Dad, Virginia and Herb, were also there with words of encouragement and love. My two older brothers, Jeff and Phil were there as well and I felt very content with all the family there, in my corner praying for me. Speaking of prayer; I believe that God hears our prayers, but you also have to wonder how many prayers are taking place at any one time and when a group is praying the same thing, that maybe that prayer may be going through to our Lord just a little louder.

The doctor came into the room and he said he had reviewed the aneurysm with his team of doctors. It turns out that he was the Chief of Staff of Ingham Hospital. He had his entire staff of eight cardiac doctors look over my heart cath. and discuss it. They had never seen anything like it and were going to have further study and discussion before surgery. I asked: "Are we going in tomorrow?" He said no, they wanted to meet some more concerning the process of addressing the aneurysm, so we would be going in on Friday. Because it was something they had never seen, they wanted to proceed with caution and start in the right spot once they had me open on the operating table. The Doctor said that this aneurysm would be a new page in the books about these cases, as there was nothing on this type to date.

So the date would be November 22nd, my older brother Jeff's birthday. The present for him on his birthday would be for his little brother to live. It was a birthday to remember, to have a successful surgery for his Lil Bro on his birthday. It also made my Mom remember, when her youngest son's surgery was on her oldest son's birthday, and just two days before her own birthday.

This time, however, I was no longer the youngster I was for my first surgery. I was 49 years old, three months short of my 50th birthday. I was in shape for a guy near half a century, but nothing near what I was at age 36. I was still lifting four to five days per week, but I wasn't doing any running anymore due to three surgeries on my right knee and two lower back surgeries since my last heart surgery.

Finally surgery morning arrived and I said "I love you" and "see you later" to Rhonda, my kids, and parents. The doctor said hello and I said "God be with you and guide your hands." I then fell off to sleep under the guidance of the anesthesiologist. I was now in the doctor's and God's hands and would not learn how things went until I woke up.

I awoke in recovery and was in and out of conscious thought. I faintly remember when the tube that was down my throat for breathing during surgery was removed. There was a slight gag response as it was pulled out but it was over quickly and I was breathing on my own. I slipped in and out of sleep and then awoke in the CICU. I had tubes and monitors attached everywhere. I had more tubes in me than orifices in my body. The largest of the tubes, once again, were the three drainage tubes coming out of my upper stomach just below my rib cage. This time, they did not merge into one, they were all separate. They were to help eliminate the fluid around the heart after surgery. One tube went around my heart and the other two went around each lung. They were about the size of a magic marker in diameter, and went down to the collector unit on the ground next to my bed.

When I awoke, my wife, kids, mom, dad, brothers and other family were there. The Doctor had already given the family the report that everything went well. So now it was time for me to start down the road to recovery again. The doctor did say that when they have to go back into a chest that has already been opened, there is a lot of scar tissue behind the sternum. It is not like the first time, where everything is clean and the cut of the sternum is quick and easy, this time they had to work their way through the scar tissue and be careful not to disturb anything that the scar tissue may have attached itself to. So that process is much, much slower, and the result is that the surgery is much longer. This one took eight hours before the report came to my wife and family.

My wife stayed in my room with me in a chair. The hospital was very helpful with extra pillows and blankets and they found her a chair that reclined, so she could lie back. I'm sure it wasn't very comfortable, but she was there for me 24/7. Those kinds of chairs are good for a few hours after a big meal and a football game on TV, but not for all night. For a couple nights she stayed at a room across the street from the hospital for patients' family members at a very reasonable rate. So check with your hospital about that possibility in your area. She was there with me throughout the whole ordeal and helped in and out of the room and helped keep my spirits up. My brothers and kids came back and forth to the hospital and my parents came back and forth many times as well. My parents delayed their annual trip to Florida until I was doing well again.

Once again, I worked through the process of the first walk. I was back in my own room again and we started through the recovery process. The first walk again with all the help just to get out of bed, the catheter, the tubes, the drainage container, medicine in a bag on a rolling rack and so on. It took a small team of people to help me up to the side of the bed and then we went for the walk and made it past the end of the bed and to the door, before starting back. The nurses were great and encouraging and cautious at the same time. They made sure I realized to save enough strength to make it back to the bed. Our first walk was in and charted and I was ready for a nap again. I improved quickly again and the next day I went for walks as often as they would let me. By the following day, my strength was up a little and they were letting Rhonda take me for my walks and things were progressing nicely. I got in contact with the interim volleyball coach who was home with my team and started talking about how practice was going and developing strategies. On the third night after surgery, Rhonda made the trip back home for the night to take care of things there. She planned to return in the morning. At 1:00 a.m., I pushed the nurses' call button, because I was having chest pains that encompassed the entire chest cavity, not just by the heart. It continued to increase, and I asked that they call Rhonda and let her know. She drove back to the hospital by around 2:30 a.m. and the pain was increasing by the minute. I have always felt that my pain tolerance was pretty high. I mentioned the many surgeries that I have had, plus all the injuries that athletes all go through.

With all the athletes that I have coached in swimming, cross country, volleyball, track and power lifting, I always used a 10-point scale for pain. One is a little owie, a stubbed toe, and 10 is so much pain, you probably need medication to help you tolerate it. My athletes knew that if their pain ever hit a six; they would not be allowed to compete or continue. If it was a five-and-a-half, they could still try, but if I saw a limp or loss of normal movement, then they had to sit and start the ICE.

Well, let's get back to me in the hospital. My pain threshold and tolerance as I mentioned was high. I was an athlete who could compete on a bloody stump and still not call it a 10. In my entire almost 50 years, I had never experienced a 10. Even after my alograft surgery on my knee, which included the removal of five years of scar tissue, and the therapist bent it until my heel touched my butt the day of surgery. But now, my whole world had crashed, because what I was feeling was a 20. What I thought was a nine in all my history, was hardly on this new scale. This new pain was incredible!

The hospital called my doctor at 2:00 a.m. and he was there by 2:30 a.m. They administered morphine to me three times in the next hour and it still wasn't taking the edge off the pain. If I can try to describe it. It felt like I had thousands of hot knives stabbing me in the entire thoracic region into my lungs from every direction. I could not move without it increasing and when they moved me to get me into the MRI, it was even worse. They transported me to the MRI room and said they would have to administer a dye to watch while in the MRI machine. Then, my wife reminded them that I might be allergic to Iodine. Of course iodine is in the dye they would use. So now the test was on hold. While waiting, I was given another shot of morphine and the pain subsided. Thank God. We did not do the MRI test and they monitored me closely for the next 24 hours and after I slept off the medicine, the pain had subsided to almost nothing. Everyone was confused, but the pain gone, so we were all ready to move on. They did keep a close watch on me to make sure if it did come back, we would be ready. That experience was the first time I really considered my longevity, as well as questioning my own pain scale. Everything I had in my head about a pain scale from one to ten was shattered; I thought I had totally lost any tolerance that I had. It was very humbling, and I had thoughts of maybe I wouldn't make it, and having wills in order and so on.

I was very impressed that my doctor had arrived so quickly in the middle of the night. Later, after I thanked him, I heard him say, "I had too much time invested into you and your special case and I wasn't going to lose you." He is why I am still here. If you remember, I secretly got his name from my catheter nurse (angel). I learned after being around him, what the nurse knew already. This Doctor will do everything in his power not to lose anyone, whether it is coming in a 2:00 a.m., working a double shift or missing his golf match. He is the type of person we all want to work on our hearts.

This experience made us all very nervous, especially my wife. She remarked that she wasn't going home again, because when she did, everything went to heck.

The next few days showed great improvement and I felt better and better each day. One thing that seemed strange was that there was one big difference for me between the two bypass surgeries that I had. If you remember, I lost a little over 20 pounds in five days after the first surgery, and that was about 4.5 pounds per day. Each day, I wanted to check my weight after the second surgery and I had lost nothing. I was still just over 200 pounds and that seemed very strange. I was pleased with the idea of when I started to get back to lifting again, that I would not have as much weight to try to regain, but at the same time, I wondered why. I have the body type of basically a tall slender guy. The only way I can gain weight is to lift weights and eat a lot. If I stop lifting, I start losing weight right away. So the fact that I had been in the hospital this long already and lost nothing was not normal for me.

The seventh night arrived and I was told that I would be going home the next day, so once again, my wife went home to get things ready for me to return home. The next morning, they took the final drainage tube out of my chest. My wife called me while she was in her one-hour drive to pick me up and she asked, "How are you doing?", and I answered, "Not too good." I felt like throwing up and my breathing started to become labored. Something wasn't right, and the pains in my chest cavity were coming back, like the ones a few nights before. She said, "I will be there as soon as I can," and she hustled her way to me.

By the time she arrived, about 45 minutes had passed and there were nurses in and out of my room as once again the knife-like pains had returned and were intensifying by the minute. Whenever I would take a breath, the pain was incredible. I felt like the only size breath I could take and tolerate the pain was about the size of a straw. If I tried to breath any more, the pain increased. My wife arrived and I knew that I didn't have much longer, but the effort to even speak was almost too much. She was scared and shocked, as everything was fine when she left the night before. What could have gone wrong, so bad, so fast?

Rhonda was on my left, and a nurse on my right. I felt myself losing the fight. It was at this time that I said a silent prayer. I asked God once again for his forgiveness of my sins, and said to him that I was coming to him and would like to be in his care, and finally that I was very anxious to reunite with my father. The nurse asked me "How are you doing?" I said, in a whisper, "I'm OK now." She asked immediately, "What do you mean, now." I spoke softly to her and said: "I have spoke to God and I am ready to go." She replied, "Not on my shift buddy."

It was then that Rhonda said to her, "What did he say?" The nurse said to me, "You tell her," and I felt so weak, I paused long enough, that the nurse repeated what I had said.

Rhonda said, "You're not going anywhere, you have too much to live for and all of us love you and the kids need you in their lives." I spoke to her and said, "I love you and tell the kids I love them but I can feel myself going." Somewhere in that time frame, I felt my eyes roll back in my head, and I really don't remember much more.

I am told that they made preparation to move me back into ICU and to get an operating room ready. They continued to try to figure out what was causing me to slip away and then the doctor spoke to Rhonda and said that all tests were showing that there was not any problem that they could nail down, but in his gut, he felt that it must be fluid build up in my chest cavity and the only way to tell was to go back in immediately. My wife, of course started to cry, and the doctor insisted. They needed her to sign some papers to allow them to go back in immediately. I remember only one thing, and that is when in the operating room, nurses moved me from my gurney to the operating table, I remember my eyes opening for a second and seeing all the lights in the room and wondering if this is the light one might see in death? My parents who had delayed their winter trip to Florida, once again delayed departure and were called back to the hospital.

The next thing I knew, I was waking up in a room that looked very strange to me. I couldn't feel the bed I was in; I could see up and peripherally, I noticed many wires and cords or cables. I couldn't see a floor and the walls appeared to be just block. I was very confused, because what I last remembered was saying goodbye. Where the heck had I ended up? I felt like I was floating or hanging from these tubes, wires and cords and a weird feeling came over me. It bothered me that there were no lights and I did not see my Dad. As I lay there, I was truly wondering; 'Where am I?' Moments later, a nurse stepped into view and said: "Welcome back, I see you're waking up." I had an internal sigh of relief come over me; My God, I had made it. They had saved me.

I still had the respirator tube in my throat, so I couldn't speak, but I realized they had figured out what was wrong and saved me. Wow, what a feeling and realization to say goodbye and then be given another chance. I used hand signals to the nurse pointing at the tube in my throat and then thumb out gesture to her, and she said: "No, we can't take it out yet, it has to stay for about another 30 minutes, and I realized I couldn't talk to find out what happened until then. I was in and out during that next 30 minutes and when it was time for it to come out, the nurse said: "OK, we are going to take the tube out now." When she removed it, I produced a fountain of vomit that came out right after the tube and I heard one of the nurses say, "Oh my", and she wiped me up immediately. The nurse told me a little about the surgery and it was shortly after that, when they let my wife come see me that she informed me what the doctors had told her.

The doctor's suspicions were right, and upon opening me back up, which this time took a mere five minutes, they found and removed two liters of fluid. This fluid which was all in my chest cavity, was taking up all the space and squeezing everything, including the lungs, which caused that pain and put so much pressure on the heart that it was having trouble beating. I'm told my blood pressure was 46/20 when they went back into my chest, as I said, my eyes had rolled back and my color was gray, with my oxygen level being very low. After removing the fluid, my vitals immediately went back to normal and during surgery, my doctor and another doctor watched my heart working for almost 30 minutes. He said, having to go back in gave him a rare opportunity to look at his work after a bypass surgery. He was able to actually lift and look over my heart and check the work he had done eight days prior. The pair of doctors watched for any seeping or leakage in the area, so they didn't close me back up right away.

Think about it. Picture a 2-liter bottle of your favorite soft drink and that is how much fluid there was in my chest cavity. I thank God for Doc as his gut feeling was exactly right, and he saved my life. They closed me back up and it was back to recovery once again.

So let us return to the room I woke up in. My wife and oldest daughter had re-contacted all of the family again and brought them up to speed on my condition. Many came to the hospital again. Most of them were certain that this was it for me. It was like I had been re-born, To see my kids, mom and dad, my brothers and many in-laws was so fantastic. They came in one at a time, to follow the hospital rules, but it was the best to see and talk to them all, and it was literally a parade of people. They all remarked about how glad they were to see me, that I made it, and don't scare the heck out of them again please. Rhonda said that my color returned immediately, when she saw me after this surgery. I was pink and looked as healthy as any time at the hospital so far. They moved me to CICU for the first night after surgery. I was back on morphine and the CICU male nurse came in and explained the timing restrictions of administering morphine and when to switch to pain pills. We talked and made the plan and I would take one more morphine prior to going to sleep, hopefully for the night, then go to the pills and if needed, maybe back to morphine after that, if the pills didn't check the pain.

That night I woke up hallucinating and caused many bells and whistles to go off in CICU, out at the nurse's station. All of a sudden, two, then three nurses were rushing into my room saying: "What's going on?" I'll tell you what was going on in my head.

My hallucination was this: I was between two bodies of water, standing on a thin peninsula of land and in each body of water to my right and left, was a speedboat. Each boat had a ski rope that was attached to my wrists and I was standing on the piece of land as the two boats hit the throttle and they were trying to drive in opposite directions. I then was forced to flex, strain and put every ounce of my strength into holding these two boats from driving apart. I was sitting up in bed with my arms outstretched in both directions groaning loudly from the strain and effort I was using to keep from getting pulled apart.

That is when the nurses came in, because they saw on their monitors, my heart rate increasing and BP going up and they heard the groans. When they came in saying, "What's going on?" I woke up and came out of the dream of hallucination. I had pulled out a few things the nurses had to redo, and I immediately stated: "No more morphine for me." I believe that the second surgery to remove fluid, while it was necessary, wasn't nearly as serious a surgery as the fixing of the bypasses and aneurysm. Because of that, I feel the morphine was too strong for what I needed and the result was that it got me all worked up. I moved out of CICU quickly, but not before I talked the nurse into giving me a shave. My father's family was from Finland, so I am a tall, blue eyed, not hairy guy, but I needed a shave. That is just an example of how good I felt already, that I felt like getting a shave and trying to clean up. I was walking circuits of the hospital the next day, as again, this emergency re-entry was just to remove fluid, which was, in and out, fairly quickly. I did however start to drop weight like a brick every day losing pounds until it was nearly 20 pounds in four days. It was because the drainage tubes were eliminating the fluid and it was not building up inside of me anymore, plus the additional interior drainage was not happening this time.

The theory of why the fluid that collected around my heart is this. The pericardium is a sack around the heart that has fluid in it that helps protect the heart with a final line of defense from a blow to the chest area. The bypass surgery removes this non-replaceable sack and people survive just fine without it. However, in a low percentage of cases, for inexplicable reasons, the body produces fluid in an attempt to fill that sack back up. The sack, of course is gone, but the body at this point has one job and that is to produce the appropriate amount of fluid in this area until a certain pressure is achieved to protect the heart. In my case, the fluid kept producing until it was virtually crushing the ability of my heart and lungs to function. This is why the doctors watched for nearly 30 minutes after removing the fluid to make sure it was not going to happen again. They saw no evidence of any more fluid being produced, so they closed me back up and we were back on the road to recovery. Thank God, and the gut feelings of my Doc.

My progress went fast the next four days in the hospital. Once the fluid was removed, I was now nine days after the bypass surgery and recovery went quickly. I was able to thank the nurse who had said: "Not on my shift, Buddy" for her efforts and insistence that I wasn't dying that day on her shift. I asked the other nurses if she was around, because I hadn't seen her after the second surgery and I wanted to thank her. I guess she had said to other nurses that she wasn't sure if I was mad at her for what she said. I assured them and her, that on the contrary, I wanted to thank her. So I found her while out on one of my walks around the circuit, and I hugged her and thanked her.

My parents waited until I was "Out of the weather" as my Mom says, and they came into my room. They were finally headed for Florida and my Mom said, "Now you go home and do what you are told, and take it easy. Your mother can't take too much more of this." I kissed Mom and Dad and said, "I am fine now, don't worry about me. You guys get down there and have a great time, and we will come down and visit you in late March, which we have been doing for the last eight years." Rhonda and I have always gone down to see them and it gave me a break between coaching volleyball and the start of the track season in the spring. So that was my plan and goal, to return to volleyball and get back to what I knew as normal.

# CHAPTER 8

## Returning Home after Second Surgery

The forth day after the second surgery, I was released and ready to get back to full recovery. My wife drove us home, and I had pillows by my chest in case of any sudden stops as an extra protection. When we arrived back home, we once again stopped by the school where my varsity volleyball team was practicing in the middle school gym. We came into the gym and the whole team ran over to the door. The players started hugging me one by one, while my wife protested and said be careful, don't squeeze him, they cut his chest open. It was great to see them as we had all been together for years of training and this was going to be my last season, and we all had goals for that season. We had several practice jerseys and the special one for that year was "50 for the Ol-Man". This shirt meant that we had to win 50 matches that season to reach one of our goals we had set as a team. We talked for a few minutes and I watched a couple minutes as they got back to their practice, and then I went home. I was pretty exhausted and went right to sleep and had a good rest for a couple of hours. They all said they were glad to see me and again lied in saying, you look good. Yea right, maybe good for a guy not dead. Next is a picture of what I had shrunk to by the time I came home.

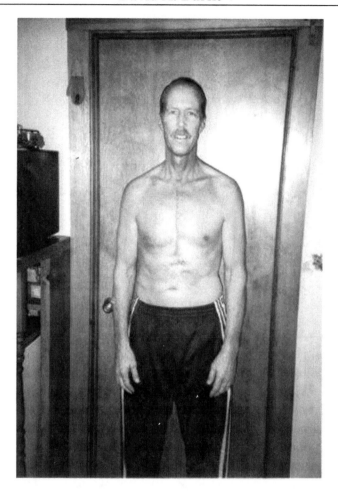

I had many visitors over the next few days and it was great to be back home. To most of my friends, the last 10 days was also a roller coaster ride. They knew I had just finished the fall cross country season, that I had had knee surgery right away so recovery would be over as much as possible before volleyball started, and maybe that I had been at the volleyball clinic, but then what most had heard was that I was in again for heart surgery, was recovering well, then almost died, had another surgery, and had made it and was now home again. It was all pretty much a surprise to everyone, because I stay in shape and look healthy. Even though they know me and my history, it's still a surprise, and it isn't something that is in their head on a daily basis, like it is in mine. I've learned to live with it and constantly know there will be another surgery, which in the current time frame should be about the year 2014. I will hold onto the prayer and hope that the medical community will come up with something by then that will be less invasive or something that acts as a draino for arteries. One can only hope.

It was colder weather this time when I got home after surgery. So I had to bundle up because of cold weather for my walks; I picked a few indoor places to walk. My best and most convenient place was to go to the school late in the evening. Most sports practices or home games were concluded by 9:00 p.m., so I would go to the school and walk at night, when the halls were clear. I would walk back and forth the length of the high school and middle school, counting the round trips to add up to a mile and then increasing distance and speed. After all, there was another treadmill test in my future. If you remember, I had knee surgery a few weeks before the heart surgery, so I was doing the physical therapy for my knee as well. I was required by the school to get a release for work from my doctor, because I wanted to return to my team as soon as I could.

The school appreciated my desire to get back to work, but also had some liability questions if I came back too soon and had a problem. I made a plan of returning to my team first, followed by half-days of teaching and my team, and finally full-time teaching and coaching. I started by going in and watching my team practice without participating at all, which as you can imagine was very tough for me. I followed the team to a Saturday tournament at the local university and watched my team and couldn't help them like I wanted to.

Within another week, in early January, I returned to coaching my team. We had a home league match that week with the toughest league opponent and made it a match, but lost. The newspaper featured a story: "Coach is Back" and ran pictures. But more important to me was the fact that we had lost. It was time to turn things up and get back on the winning track. Coincidentally, the match that night was against Sir, the coach/friend I had attended the volleyball clinic with back in November when I had the attack, which led to finding the aneurysm.

It was great being back, and it was unfortunate to be up against my friend's tough program the first match back, but it also was kind of a neat coincidence. The team was glad to have me back and that felt good, too. School was still out for Christmas break, so it worked out well for me to return to practices first. Once school started after the break, I started that first week with half-days and practice after school or matches. In my absence, the team had 12 wins to six losses and three splits. For the rest of the season we were 29-12-4 for a total of 41 wins for the season. That was short of our goal of 50 for that year, but we had quite a season. As planned prior to the season, this would be my last season of coaching volleyball.

I returned to school and coaching as you know, but I was in need of others to help with many things throughout the day. I still couldn't lift over 10 pounds of anything, and I was teaching weight training in three classes per day. My other two hours were middle school art and yearbook, both easy physically, but I still had to rely on others for moving things when necessary. Plus, the yearbook assignment was a high stress position with deadlines every day. When volleyball was over and track started, I was getting stronger and able to lift more, but still not what I was used to. Moving equipment in track and field many times deals with heavy equipment, like Pole Vault pits, hurdles; even the boxes and tubs of uniforms were too heavy. The writing of workouts and verbally coaching the athletes went fine, but not being able to physically do all I wanted to do was very frustrating to me. I used to throw the discus, and I wanted to do it all again. I had to consider slowing down, even though I loved coaching, and I had already decided that the previous volleyball season would be my last. With my history of being a type A personality and striving hard always to win, and be the best, this was a difficult consideration to start thinking of something less physical and stressful. But for the time being, I worked hard at holding my own and keeping up the front that everything was fine.

# 50<sup>th</sup> Birthday

My wife surprised me with a huge 50<sup>th</sup> birthday party in March, about four months after surgery and about a month after my actual birthday. That's why it was such a surprise. Volleyball season is typically over in early March. Rhonda planned out a party in a banquet room of a local bar/restaurant. We tend to have Friday night dinners at this establishment quite often, so it didn't seem strange that we were going there again on a Friday night. We walked in through the back door and saw some people at the first table that I knew and we started talking. The banquet room was off to the side, away from where we entered, and I heard later that my brother was in the front of that bar section when I walked in the back door, but I didn't see him duck back into the banquet room.

We took a seat at the bar while we waited for a table (or so I thought) and I put our name in for a table for four. A few minutes later, the bar owner who knew that I was the supervisor of the yearbook at the school cleverly came up to me and started a conversation about some old pictures that he had found of our home town and would I like to see them. Always working or doing something related to the school or my team, I agreed to walk next door to see these pictures. He took me to the banquet room, which was dark. He didn't turn on the light and backed up and said the pictures are spread out on the first table, and motioned for me to go in. That seemed strange, but I was still clueless and walked in. The lights came on and there was about 75 people in there who all yelled "Surprise!" I was in total shock as I looked around the room and saw people from all aspects of my life. I was still confused as to why all these people were here. I knew they had all just yelled surprise, but they couldn't be there for me. It took a few moments to sink in. I started to actually make eye contact with people around the room and wave and nod and say hi. I don't know if it was because I just had the surgery or what, but as I looked at everyone around the room, each time I focused on someone it seemed like they represented a different chapter from my life. There were, of course family from both my side and Rhonda's side, there were former students, there were former athletes, people from the health clubs that I had owned, coaches, staff members, and administrators from school, coaches I competed against, my Macker partner, people I lifted with and competed against and more. It was all very moving for me, to think that they would all come, and that my wife had pulled off such a surprise.

We spent about three hours there with food, drinks, and conversation and laughs and I had a great time, and I have complimented Rhonda many times for pulling it off without me knowing a thing. It was just what I needed at that time.

You know you have friends and you get busy with things, but it's nice to have an outward sign like that. It was a real boost to me.

Schools take a week-long spring break around March and Rhonda and I were accustomed to traveling down to Florida where my parents have a condo in the panhandle. We flew this time, just to make it easier on both of us. I have always been one of those marathon drivers and drive straight through, and Rhonda would prefer to stop part way, so we compromised by flying, which also doubled as a trip with no travel stress. It was a great week of relaxation and it couldn't have come at a better time. We did absolutely nothing except go to bed late, get up late, walk the beach, nap on the beach, go out for dinners and have a couple evenings out. It was a very calming 10 days.

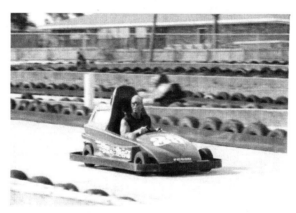

I then returned to school and the normal day-to-day stress that comes up with classes, coaching the track team, and striving to win. Throw in some new personal stress and I knew it was time to change paths. That year was to be my last in the public school system and I retired in June. While it added stress to leave what I loved, it also lifted a huge workload that was tougher than before.

I set in motion the sale of our rental duplex, which we owned and operated. A few months later, it sold and we paid off many bills and eliminated yet two more sources of stress. With the rental sale and paying off some bills, all we had was our house payment and, for us, a fat bank account. I say, fat for us, because we have always been on a check-to-check budget, with little savings. We had all we needed and were doing fine, but there was no nest egg, as they call it, and now we had a little one.

## Returning To Lifting And Staying In Shape Again

I was teaching weight training at the High School, so it was pretty convenient to start lifting again as soon as I was able. I starting lifting within 3 weeks, very light at first and then slowly increased my weights to start to build again. After lifting weights for so long, I didn't like being so skinny. Muscles have a good memory and respond well to getting back to work and rebuild. I trained 4 and 5 days per week, and still train to date 4 days per week. My son, who was in Colgate was training hard and when he was home, I love training with him. Back in the day, he wasn't strong enough to even spot the weights I was using, and now he out lifts me regularly, that's the way it should be, and I am so proud of him.

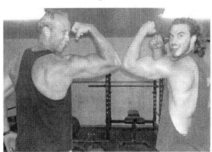

*Showing off with my son Erik*

## Retired From Teaching

In June of 2002, I retired from the public school System after 28 years of service, having taught and coached swimming in the early years, taught in the middle school, physical education, history, math, earth and life science, journalism, and art. Then later, in the high school, I taught physical education, weight training and yearbook. I was honored to be included in the "Who's Who Among America's Teachers" eight times, three times honored as An Outstanding Professional from an area university. In the varsity sports arena, my teams accomplished victory for the home team over 1,000 times. More than half of all those victories were after the first heart surgery. I was honored with "Statewide Coach of the Year" three times, Regional Coach of the Year many more times, League championship teams over a dozen times. Hundreds of my athletes went on to compete in college, many on scholarships, and many went on to coach others, some of them at schools where they were against me in competition. In power lifting, we accomplished wins in seven state championships, were national champs once and runner up another year. I trained and coached many individual state champions, four national champions, a world champ and a runner up in the world. I also trained many bodybuilders, a few accomplished state titles and some in national competition. I also owned and operated four different health clubs for a 10-year period in the middle of my school years. I had a lot to be happy about, but it was time to move onto something less stressful, and stop and smell the roses, as they say. After everything that had happened, I knew I could not carry on in the way that I needed to work and coach, and life would not be the same, and I had to make a decision.

## Building My New Home

In October of 2003, my wife and I purchased some land. We used the balance of what was left after we sold our rental duplex and had paid off all our bills. The land was three-quarters of an acre and I immediately started clearing the land of all what was left there. There was a tragic situation that had occurred on the property and the land eventually came up for auction. It was covered with things that were hard to even fathom. Those who remember the show "Sanford and Son" will have an idea of what was on the land, from a 1972, 70-foot mobile home grown in by 15 trees, plus nine sheds and lean-tos full of only what I can call, stuff. There were chicken coops, cement chunk piles, fence pieces, rock piles, woodpiles and thick underbrush covering the entire three-quarters of an acre. I spent the next three months seven days a week, at my pace, cleaning, clearing, burning, recycling, trashing, and selling the metal. I felt if I just finished cleaning and clearing the land, we could sell the lot for more than what we had paid for it, or continue into building a new home.

During that time, during our travels, we started searching out and looking at homes we liked. In time, we designed our home with all the things we liked and wanted. I made a rough drawing of what we wanted, with dimensions and then hunted for someone to blueprint it. Next, I started talking to builders to rough or frame it in. We chose a group to rough it in and we broke ground for the walk out basement in December of 2003. The framers were done with the rough in by mid January. Living in Michigan, I had to actually shovel snow out of the house twice before the roof went on, I even used the snow blower to remove snow from the house. It looked done from the outside, and then it was time for me to start inside.

I had continued work outside on the land while the framing was taking place. I then started inside and worked steadily, first with the furnace and heating system, then plumbing and electric, and I finished all the work within the walls. Then all the extra framing for our special features, such as tri-ceiling in the kitchen, raised counter framing, because we are tall, radius framing for some circle drywall in corners in the recreation room, interior window framing for a stained glass window, wiring the 23-foot cathedral ceiling for special fans, skylights in a cathedral ceiling in an interior upstairs master bathroom, and more. Then it was blow-in insulation time, drywall, painting, cupboards, trim work and lighting. I worked steadily for the next 10 months in order to finish. I put in the hard wood floors, tiled the bathrooms and walk-in shower, added drop ceilings in additional bedrooms and got the house ready for us to move into it by the week before Christmas of 2004. We celebrated our first Christmas here in 2004. I then finished the clearing of what remained outside and leveled the entire lot to make a nice lawn. Exterior landscaping was a continuous project for the next 4 years, with field stones and cut steps into a clay hill behind the house, next to the walk out basement. I also had constructed a 10' by 16' screened in gazebo and ran electric out to it, and included and patio and fire pit. It is great to see deer walk through the back yard, and wild turkey, rabbits and some visitors that are not welcome. The final touch was the ash fault circle driveway out front. I had to cap off a well as the house is plumbed to the City sewer and water, as the front is within the village limit and the back section is in the township, giving the option of raising wildlife and have campfires, which is a great combination. I saved thousands of dollars building it myself and figured out that I could mess up an area 5 times before it would be the same price as hiring someone to do it. I made sure that I did it right the first time, and developed a good relationship with inspectors, and I really wanted to do it right and they knew that and appreciated it.

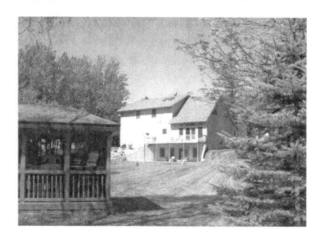

# CHAPTER 9

## Sexual

L et's be frank about this area. No one wants to talk about how they are affected, but it is a simple comparison that if the blood vessels in your heart are clogged and the blood flow is restricted, that it is also restricted in your penis. The blood vessels in your penis are just as susceptible to clogging as the ones by your heart, and when they do, your erection is going to be affected.

Many people will notice an erectile change and not know what it means. Erectile change is an early clue to you that restricted blood flow is occurring. Most men will not say a word when they first notice a change. It may be a simple change at first. You may not be able to hold an erection as long as you used to. But it is easy at this point to write it off to a normal occurrence of getting older. You may be in a sexual encounter and lose your erection during intercourse. Your partner may be saying, "That's OK", but really be thinking, "Is it me, does he not want to be with me, do I not turn him on?" Or any such questions to herself or to you. The answer may be both simple and complex. You may simply have restricted blood flow in your penis in the early stages of clogging arteries. While you should be rejoicing that you have been given a clue that a problem in clogging is underway, instead, you are disappointed in yourself, embarrassed, upset, and trying to explain something you have little control over, or ability to explain; because it is clogging that is causing it.

You may have already been aware of a heart problem and your doctor has put you on medication that has a side effect of impotency. Many medications, while they lower your blood pressure very well, have a beta-blocker in them, which will result in loss of erection. Many men at this point would choose death. That may sound ignorant, cruel, or stupid, but if you ask a hundred men, "If we give you a pill which will make you live longer, but your penis may not work." Most will say. "Keep your pill, I'd rather die with a hard on, than live and not be able to get one." Don't despair, keep trying the different medications with your doctor's help until you find the one that lowers your BP and doesn't have side effects. You have to lighten up on yourself with things that you don't have control of, and talk about it with your doctor and your partner. You will have a lot less stress and let's face it, stress adds to this high BP problem. High BP and stress add to restricting of arteries and consequently clogging occurs quicker, so the vicious circle begins and gets worse for you.

Beta Blockers block the chemical or hormonal messages sent to the heart. When you are under physical or emotional stress, your body sends signals to your heart to work harder. Beta-blockers block the effect these signals have on your heart, so they reduce the amount of oxygen your heart demands. One side effect of these beta-blockers is erectile dysfunction, or the failure to sustain an erection.

Calcium channel blockers can help to keep your arteries open and reduce your blood pressure by relaxing the smooth muscle that surrounds the arteries in your body. The oxygen demand of the heart is also reduced by these medicines.

## EDM

When it becomes necessary, your doctor may prescribe Erectile Dysfunction Medication, or EDM. Your Doctor may prescribe 50 or 100 mg tabs to help with circulation. EDM will help you to lead a close to normal sex life and reduce stress. Both of you can enjoy sexual activity and reduce the anxieties of erectile dysfunction.

You and your partner will still have to develop a healthy attitude about the use of EDM. EDM works a little differently for all people.

You may experience results from the pill 60 minutes after taking it, or it might be 30 or 75 minutes. You will have to experiment with it and find out for yourself. Taking the EDM on a full stomach will change the effectiveness of it. You will find that sexual intercourse will be a planned situation; due to the fact that you will need to take your pill a certain number of minutes before the act will be successful, and not too close after a big meal. This takes away the spontaneity of sex. Once again, you will need a partner who is on board with you in this regard. It changes the psyche of the impending encounter. If you have trouble coming to terms with this planning and decision process, it will be another source of stress. So try to communicate with your partner and come to some sort of agreement so that both parties don't feel uncomfortable, forced or coerced into an activity that should be glorious for both of you, or, as I said, it will add stress, and we know that restricts blood flow, raises blood pressure and causes more heart problems.

A lot of people have a tough time talking about their penis, because of its private nature. The penis is simply a body part that has two functions, one being to urinate and the other to have intercourse and ejaculate, so I am going to consider the penis simply as a part of the body and treat it that way. EDM helps with that second task, when the penis is working properly; ejaculation is a four-step process with arousal, erection, stimulation and ejaculation. Sound simple? With many men, step two does not happen, eliminating step 3 and 4. He may be stimulated, but there is no erection. What is the technology of an erection? First, remember, when you want to move a body part, you do it using muscle, you think about it and contract the muscle and that body part moves. Your penis is completely different. Like a balloon, when you put air in it, it gets larger and harder. Your penis needs blood to the proper pressure to accomplish that same goal, an erection. The penis has two cigar shaped structures called corpora cavernosa that it uses to become erect. If a person's blood flow is restricted due to clogging, the process of filling the corpora cavernosa to the right pressure will not occur. EDM helps in this blood flow. The average male has 4-8 erections per night during REM sleep. A doctor can actually fit the penis with a sensor to see whether you are having erections during REM. If you are not, then you probably have a blockage and an EDM may be prescribed for you. If you are achieving erections during REM, then your physical system is working properly, and your erectile dysfunction may be psychological, or a combination of both. You may then find yourself in a situation where you are stressed out about your ability to get an erection, which then works against your ability to get one.

## Possibility Of Disability

This is an avenue you might want to look into. You may still feel like you want to take on the world, but after all you have been through you may have to face it. You just can't do what you used to be able to do. The retirement system of the job you have been doing may have some answers for you. If you are in a situation now, after your surgery, that you cannot do what you used to, contact your human resources department and find out what you might be qualified for or entitled to. If you are able to return to your job and continue what you were doing, then you have recovered well and more power to you. However, you may have to consider that you cannot continue in the manner you were before and then it's nice to know your options. It may be a complete career change will solve the problem of not being able to physically do what you did before. If you qualify for disability, there will be forms to fill out and doctors to verify things, but the result may be receiving compensation for the years of service you have worked up until this point. Check into these things, so you don't add stress, because we know what that does to hearts, don't we?

# CHAPTER 10

## Family And Friends, What To Expect

This section is written from information gathered from others who were around and witnessed my heart surgeries. Their view was from the other side of the bed. It might help you to understand what others may be going through during a surgery. These are all family and great friends whom I love very much and thank God they were there for me then and still now. The following are some of their thoughts, concerns, and observations.

My mother said that when she heard that I was going in for the first open heart surgery, she was very apprehensive. I had already had many surgeries, but nothing as serious as this. She says: I knew David would be very positive about his ability to recover, and he knew that he had the support and love of the whole family. As far as my expectations of how David would do, I knew he would do well. David was never afraid, as far as we knew; he said and felt if things didn't go right, that he would be with his father. I simply gave it all up to God and knew He would be guiding the doctor's hands. After the surgery, David never treated himself as an invalid. David's ability to do as directed and even more cut his recovery time in half.

Then years went by and we got news of his second surgery, and I thought, 'Not again,' but I still remained very hopeful. Going into this one, I knew that David would be very positive again, as he always dealt with any adversity in his life. Who knows what is really going on inside anyone else, but he once again stayed strong and seemed to stay very positive. Things were progressing according to plan, and then we received the news that he had to go back in. This is when I thought, My God, I'm going to lose my baby! From the time David was born, he had so many things go wrong, and he had so many surgeries, I always had the feeling that he was just on loan to me for a short time, and how he was being taken away from me. I was scared during this part and I did a lot of talking to God and the whole family. David started to work right away to recover and when he asked the doctor if there were going to be any restrictions, I know David didn't want to hear any. He didn't go through this ordeal to be told he couldn't do what he wanted to do with his life.

My Stepfather, Dad, as I call him had these thoughts: My concern right away was that he had inherited a heart problem from his birth father and grandfather. I anticipated that David would pull through, but that he would have to slow down, and that would be very hard for him to do. Once he recovered, he had pulled through fine, but he didn't slow down. But, that's David. I was very concerned because of his past health history and that he was having a five-way bypass at the age of 36. After surgery, I was amazed at his speedy recovery and the way he pushed himself. I always admired Dave's determination to get the job done. Once he set his course, he just would not quit. He handled this problem and his recovery in a manner way beyond what I expected.

When we heard about him going in for the second surgery, I had the same concerns, but multiplied from the first one. Now he was nearly 50years old. I still felt that he would pull through fine, and again felt he would have to slow down. My expectations of him recovering were correct at first, as he was doing fine and we left the hospital in high spirits because he was doing so well. We planned to continue with our original plans of going to Florida for the winter. Then we heard he was going back into surgery, and I was deeply shocked and concerned for his mother. I was afraid that his mother's feeling that she was losing him was going to happen. I wanted to shield her as much as I could. Once he was out of surgery and doing so much better, we were relieved and eventually headed for Florida as planned. David shows what a positive attitude and determination can do. You have to push yourself. His way is the way to go.

My wife had only heard about the first surgery and knew that there was another one coming at some point. When I felt pain at the volleyball clinic and came home, I didn't tell her about it, because I wondered if the pains were due to the medication that I was taking for the rash by my knee, after that surgery. I really hoped that by me not taking it anymore, the pain might not hit me again. I was wrong, and Monday morning, when I excused myself from school, I called her at work and informed her about it. Then she got worried, came home and we went to the hospital to get checked out. Next was my cardiologist visit, and then the scheduled heart catheterization in Lansing. That was when I first learned that we were not going home, and they were admitting me right away. She was then told while I was still hooked up for the heart cath. The doctors told her what was going on, in the next room from me, and I could see them behind a glass wall. The following are her thoughts.

I was stunned, and didn't want to do this, but knew we had to go through it. It was all new to me, and so overwhelming as they explained things to me and things happened so fast, there was no time to prepare. It was out of work Monday, cardiologist Tuesday, heart cath Wednesday, admitted into the hospital the same day and surgery was scheduled. There was no time to think or plan. I didn't want to go through it, but had to be strong and take one day at a time.

I felt good about Dave's chances. He is positive, healthy, and he's a fighter. My expectations eventually became reality; he was doing good for a while, and the minute I went home on the fourth night, then suddenly he couldn't breathe and had terrible chest pains. I thought right away that the tubes in his chest were coming out too early, because there was still a lot of fluid draining, and the first of the tubes had come out that day. I hurried back to the hospital as fast as I could get there. I walked into the room and he looked terrible. He was white and sweaty and having a terrible time breathing, and then I was really scared. That night was when the doctor came in at 2:30 a.m. and they ran all kinds of tests and shot Dave up with morphine again., They still didn't figure out what caused the pain and breathing trouble, but it subsided. So then, I felt that I had to stay at the hospital to be an advocate and take care of him.

We were treated great and the care was great, but that fluid still coming out of his chest and then removing the first tube really bothered me. Plus he had to urinate about every 15 minutes, so often that I was emptying his bedside urinal over and over. He was filling it so often and pushing the nurse button for them to empty it again, that I just started emptying it myself. One night they gave him a diuretic to help him get rid of fluids, because the chest tubes were still flowing, and then he had to go every five minutes. There was no sleeping that night.

Another night, about 10:00 p.m., I was in Dave's room with him and we both heard some commotion in the hall. I could see right out the door and down the hall and suddenly a man in his mid-50s, naked as the day he was born, comes running down the hall straight towards our room. Right after him, there were two nurses right on his heels. He came so fast, I didn't even have time to try to close our door and he was in our room and started towards Dave's bed still running. That was very strange, his meds had him out of his head or something, and so we kept our door closed after that.

Things were improving again and the last tube came out, again before I thought it should, because fluid was still draining but it was normal that by this day after surgery, the tubes come out. I went home again and by the time I got back to take him home the next morning, he couldn't breathe again and the pain was back and worse than before. Then I got scared again. They ran all kinds of tests and couldn't figure it out. All the tests, scans for clots, x-rays, they found nothing wrong, but he was getting weaker and weaker. Sometime during that morning, Dave felt himself fading and said Goodbye to me I told him he had too much to live for to talk like that. They were shooting him up with morphine again every 30 minutes to try to stop the pain. The Doctor finally came to me and said, he had to open Dave back up, and that he had a feeling that Dave was filling with fluids, and nothing else was showing up. He was already back in ICU and I told the Doctor to do what was best. Then I started praying and calling the family. I didn't see him for three and a half hours after that. Then family members were showing up during that time. We finally heard that the doctor's gut feeling was right and they removed two liters of fluid from his chest. He was in recovery and I could go see him. Shortly after that, they let the family back to see him, two at a time. His daughters, mom and dad, brothers and many from my family all took their turns to go see him. We then were told that they needed to bathe him, because during this ordeal, he had done a lot of sweating, and he needed some rest. Two more hours went by before I saw him again and when I saw him, he was pink, and looked healthier than he had looked the whole time he had been in there. It was a huge relief and I knew he was on the road to recovery.

Nothing about this whole thing was normal. He was the exception to all the rules in recovery. He would seem to be doing good and then something would go wrong. When he had lower back surgery, they left bone spurs in, and that caused problems. They had to go back in and file down the spurs. Because he is younger than most patients going through heart surgery and he seems to recover well, they tend to send him home too early, and it doesn't always happen that way for him. From my experience, I would have someone there in the hospital with the patient, learn the medication time schedule and what they are taking and when, bring a pillow and blanket and stay and be there for them. Don't take things for granted. If you're there, you can help keep track of things, even if it's for your own peace of mind. Trust your doctor. I need to say that everyone was so helpful, Dave just wasn't following the norm. Trust your judgment, I feel, plan on staying for the long haul, that way you will be there if something comes up.

My oldest daughter, Crandall, my Rock, has followed in my footsteps of being organized and the "Get the job done" girl. She is soft as they come, or she can put the fear of God in you with a glance, and everything in between. I've always told her: "I am the first man ever to have loved you and the one who will never take that love away from you."

These are her thoughts: When my father had his first open heart surgery I was only twelve years old. I was not told a lot and have limited memories about that time. I do remember everyone at school asking me about how he was doing since I was attending the middle school where he taught. At the hospital they told me that he would be full of tubes and kept telling me not to be scared or get upset. To tell you the truth, if they would have just said he will have some tubes but he is ok that would have been less scary. Everyone really tried to keep my life as normal as possible. My grandmother stayed with us for about a month and helped dad take care of me.

In 2002, for Dad's second surgery, I was living in Northern Michigan and was busy climbing the corporate ladder. My dad called telling me about the chest pains that he had over the weekend and that he was going to have some tests run. At this point he said that there was no need to worry and that he would let me know when everything was taken care of. He had some routine tests and they decided that he needed to have a heart cath. to see what was going on. I remember talking to him the day before the heart cath. Let me tell you a little something about my dad. Whenever anything like this comes up he is determined to make sure that you are not worried and he spends most of his energy putting your mind at ease. He is more focused on the fact that you should not worry than he is on letting you know he may be worried himself.

Even when he said that they were headed to the hospital to have the heart cath the following morning he was telling me not to worry. He was so sure that there would be something small and that it could be taken care of quickly. The following day I was just getting ready to leave for work when I got the message from Rhonda that they were keeping him in the hospital. They were going to have to open him up again. My world crashed down around me as I listened to her words.

There I was three hours away from him and feeling like I could not get there fast enough. I wanted to get in my car right then and leave but I knew that I had to get my brother who was still at school. I have a hard time remembering the timing of everything that happened in the next hour. I was so upset by everything and scared that I was going to lose my father. I needed to leave as fast as I could and was frantic to get to him. Because I was so upset it was decided that someone would drive me to Lansing. My brother would follow with my mother later that evening and they would come to Lansing the next day. I have to tell you, that was the longest three hours I have ever driven. All I kept thinking was that the world needed to stop until I saw my dad.

As soon as I saw him I felt better. He did not look sick at all and that can be deceiving. I started to worry less and got down to the business of "what is the plan of attack?" Of course, you know where

I learned that from. OK, this is where we are and now let's make the best of it. We had just been handed lemons and we both decided to make lemonade. We started to talk about what needed to be done with school and coaching. Having played four years on Dad's varsity team and having been a volleyball coach myself I knew that he needed to take care of his team. Once we knew that we had one more day before the surgery, we got a list of things that I needed to get from the house and school for him.

I went home to the house that I grew up in. I have to say that it was a very lonely feeling being there by myself for the night. I finally was able to let down and was overcome with the fear of losing my father. I knew that we would be doing this surgery again but I was still not prepared. What would we do if we lost him? The next day I headed back to the hospital with everything. We worked most of the afternoon and after that I had a lot of plans to take back to the school for his classes and his team. Being able to do that made it feel like I still had a measure of control over something, and that I was helping Dad.

Into surgery he went and all we could do was wait. That was a very long day. One of the things that my dad may not even realize is how much he brought my family together that day. Having divorced parents is never easy but we had managed to make our way through pretty well. As children you now have "two" families. My mother and stepmother were there waiting together, both for very different reasons. My mother, not wanting to lose the father of her children and my stepmother not wanting to lose her husband. Grandparents and uncles were there, all of whom had not been in the same room in too many years. We were all there together, and we created and renewed bonds all because of my father.

We got the word that he was out of surgery and in CICU. He looked pretty out of sorts but he was still with us. We were now on the road to recovery. I really don't remember how fast he recovered from the first surgery so I thought that he was doing well. He did seem to be very uncomfortable but everyone said that was normal. The next days went by pretty fast and I headed back to work with my dad on the mend and counting the days to going home. I kept my phone on me at all times and made sure that I was kept up to date on his progress. Then I got a call from my stepsister saying that he was going back into surgery. I called the school and they had my brother waiting outside when I picked him up. I cannot imagine the worry that he must have felt knowing that something very wrong was happening. I do not know how long it took us to get there but I should probably have gotten a few tickets along the way.

Now this surgery was different and we were all scared that he may not make it out of it. I knew that he had made peace with God and that he was ready to be with his father. I can tell you that I told God that he could not have him yet and that he would have to wait. We needed him here a whole lot longer. He is the first man that loved me and I was not about to let him go.

When I got to see him after the surgery he looked great. He looked better than he had any of the eight previous days. He had great color and was in high spirits. He looked like he had a weight lifted off him as he quite literally had. I was able to stay with him one of his nights in the hospital so that Rhonda could get home and take care of things on that end. I can tell you that the chair was not that comfortable but I survived and the nurses really tried to make me feel at ease. It was hard to watch him try to sleep in such discomfort. He had to do breathing exercises and walks around the halls. It was quite a sight to watch this mountain of a man have trouble breathing deeply. He has been like a superhero to me since I was a little girl. It is hard to watch someone you love struggle with things we take for granted like breathing.

For a while after the surgery my father looked at least ten years older than he had just two weeks before that. That Christmas we celebrated the gift of having him there with us. He now looks younger than his age and still acts like a youngster even though his body is starting to remind him that he is a senior citizen. I know that we will have to do this surgery again and we will approach that just like we do every other thing. Prepare, plan, organize and get ready to start recovering when it is done.

When I think about if he had not made it through either of those surgeries it makes me sad. He would have missed so many things. He never would have seen my sister graduate college or my brother graduate high school. He would not have been there to walk me down the aisle or hold his first granddaughter. Every day that we have with him is a blessing.

My 2$^{nd}$ daughter, Malissa, the care taker, giver, and passionate athlete. Whenever anyone needs comforting, she is there with genuine caring.

My daddy has arms I swung from as a child. He is a father who isn't afraid to cry and is so proud of his children.

When I was eight he was taken to the hospital. I remember not really knowing what was going on. But my grandmother came to stay with my sister, brother and I while my mom went with him. I was so angry that no one was telling me what was really going on because I was so young. Now I have to admit I was an old eight-year-old and really thought all my questions should be answered. I was so scared but at eight I thought nothing could bring down this mountain of a man. We went to East Grand Rapids to see him and I was not prepared. He was in bed and just looked too tired. I remember feeling like he was just sick and would be all right. I saw in his eyes that he knew himself he would be ok, I knew not to think anything different.

Throughout the rest of my childhood I learned more about the history of heart disease in my family. My father continued to have his "routine" stress tests and we knew ten years down the road there would probably be a need for another surgery. Ten turned into 11, into 12, and I thought everything would be all right.

I was a junior in college at Colgate University when my father called me. He called to say that he was going in for a different type of test this time because of his recent knee surgery. He said not to worry, that everything would be all right and that he would call me the following day; again I couldn't think anything different. I am not sure who he was convincing that day, me or himself?

The next morning I got up and went to class. I had a full day of classes and meetings, followed by lunch and then directly to basketball practice. I walked into practice late, running from class and my two best friends/teammates/roommates and my head coach started to walk towards me. They seemed like they were in slow motion and the look on their faces sent chills up my spine. Once they reached me I just kept saying "What, tell me now, what?" They took me into the coaches' office and told me that my family had been calling all day (this was a pre-cell phone era), and that my father was having to go in for emergency open heart surgery.

I felt like the room was spinning and felt so scared. I didn't know really what that meant, other than I had to get home as soon as possible. My team's opening game was in two days and I knew I would have to miss it. Luckily the NCAA has a program for family emergencies and they were able to buy me a plane ticket home the next morning.

I got to the hospital the next day and walked in to talk to my dad. He was up on two feet laughing and visiting with my family. There was my dad, smiling like he always is and enjoying his time with my family regardless of what was to follow. He hugged me and told me he was going to be all right and not to worry. I knew again to trust him but still felt anxious and scared.

The following day he went in for his surgery. The wait felt like forever and I felt myself snapping at my family out of my own frustration and stress. He came out of surgery fine and was in ICU when I finally got to see him. He had tubes coming from his chest and a tube down his throat. His blue eyes gave me peace when they locked with mine. He was there and he was present in that room after surgery. He was not very responsive, but I held his hand and said my "I love you." I remember standing outside the room watching my family go in one by one and see my dad. I will always remember when my Uncle Phil went in to see his brother. My dad had been there staring up, but still looked defeated. When Uncle Phil went in, my dad lit up. There was no question that what my uncle was saying was giving my dad strength. He grasped his hand and nodded his head. This was something that he hadn't done with anyone else in the room. My uncle gave my father strength that day, strength only a brother can give and a brother can understand. I stood there next to my brother and sisters and felt the same. My sister's hand was brushing lightly on my back and my brother was holding my hand. My father gave us that same gift. It will always be the gift that gives me strength and was shown to me on that day that it can never be replaced.

Everything seemed to be progressing as planned and he was on his way to recovery. My cousin drove me back to New York so that I could tie up lose ends with my professors and play in my team's second basketball game of the season. I drove in the day of the game and was still able to play. The next day the team and I left for Buffalo to play a game right before Thanksgiving. After our game I got a ride back to Michigan and back to my father. I sat in the room with my dad as he ate his Thanksgiving dinner and listened to him breathe. He had slowed in his recovery and kept saying that he wasn't feeling so great.

His blood pressure was dropping and he was having a really hard time taking in deep breaths. I saw in his eyes that he was hurting. On a scale from one to ten, any normal person's ten would be my father's five in terms of pain. When he said his pain was an eight to the nurse, I knew whatever was going on inside of him was serious. He told me that he had spoke to his deceased father and was ready to go. I told him to hold on and that I loved him. He told me how proud of me he was and that he loved the woman I was becoming. The doctor was called in and after checking on him decided that his blood pressure was dropping so quickly that he had to go back in and find out what was happening.

I think that I was prepared to have him go in the first time, but the second time, I was not. I didn't understand what was going on, what could possibly be going so wrong inside of him and why he didn't continue to feel better like he had before. This time was much quicker and the doctor came out right away to tell us that fluid had been building up around his heart and slowly compressing it, slowing his heartbeat and essentially killing him. He assured us that he was all right and that he was glad he went back in. From then on things seemed to get better. After this surgery he continued to get better and got out of the hospital in a normal amount of time. I saw my dad again over Christmas and he was up on his feet again, but slow. He looked much older than he did the day that I walked into the hospital room before his first surgery. But the fight in my father was still fierce. He started to push the envelope and started to lift slowly again after he was cleared. His coloring started to come back and today he looks great. My father's arms might even be bigger than when I was a little girl. I am sure that he could tell you the exact measurements to this day.

My father is so special to my family and me. He got to walk his first child down the aisle and was there when his first grandbaby was born. He got to see me graduate college and has continued to be my support and shoulder to cry on. My daddy's arms carry so much, they carry my love, my family, my strength and my hope that no matter what, my daddy's steel-blue eyes will always be proud of me.

My son Erik, I worry about the most; that maybe he has inherited my bad genetics and clogging heart. The last thing I want him to get from me is clogging in his heart. What I do know is that he has a loving, caring heart. Don't get me wrong, I have never blamed my genetics on my Dad and I know that if he had a chance, he too would express the same feelings of not wanting to pass that trait onto his kids. I know there is nothing anyone can do about it, but I still think about it. One thing I believe in is a statement I heard many years ago. "Don't waste time with worry. God stays up all night worrying, so we don't have to."

The following is from Erik: My father, Dad, or Pops, as I call him, had his first surgery when I was only three, so I really have no recollection of it, but his second one was when I was a junior in high school. It was a normal day at school and I was told that my Mother had called and was coming to pick me up early. I was scared from the beginning, without ever being told what it was; I knew something must be wrong; I could feel it. Immediately, I thought of Dad for some reason. I stood in the parking lot waiting for Mom and I cried. I was told later what was going on, but I was confident that he would make it through. I had an eerie calm about the way I approached the whole situation. I never doubted Dad, I never thought he had a chance to die, he was too strong. He'd been through it before, he could do it again. Maybe it was my naivety or sheer denial, but something in me told me not to worry. My expectations eventually came to pass, as I knew they would; he was just too strong to lose.

When I heard he was going back in again eight days later for surgery, I was angry at first, with the doctors and life in general, but I was ready to give my support and love at a moment's notice. This time, doubt had crept into my mind. I thought, wow, he could really go at this point, so I tried to think of deep meaningful things to say, but all I could say is, "I Love You." Which I think gets the point across. My thoughts that my father could be gone this early into my life, I thought of things like: He hasn't seen me through college, and that he wouldn't be able to watch me on the field ever again, or he'd never meet my wife, or see his only son have children of his own. I've always wanted to meet Edwin, Dad's Dad, so I want my kids to know Pops.

As far as his recovery, I don't recall too much, but what I do remember from that time, was how old Dad looked. He usually weighed 210 pounds, 20 to 25 pounds more than me, and now I'm out weighing him by like 10-15 pounds, that's never happened before. But I was surprised how fast the recovery time was, he was back to normal very fast (faster than I expected) and life was even sweeter since then.

My daughter Erin was adopted prior to my 2nd surgery, and I was married to her mom by that time. She said: My initial thoughts were that Dad was having an extensive surgery, but I knew that he would come out of it fine, because he is a fighter. I expected him to do well with the surgery and I never started to really worry until after the bypass surgery and I visited him in the ICU. My expectations of him coming out well all changed when he got worse and had to go back into surgery or he would have died.

That's when things got scary for me. At that time, when he went back in for another surgery, I don't know what I thought. There were so many emotions running through my head, all I knew is that I was scared. Then I was just nervous, scared and very emotional. When he was recovering, I was driving back and forth from where I lived to visit and I didn't see a lot of his recovery; it is all kind of a blur to me. I know it took awhile, but this was a very stressful and emotional time for me, so the actual time line is difficult to remember. My advice to others is to keep your head up and try to stay positive and it's nice to have friends and family around.

I think you can see why I am so proud of my kids. They can make me smile with a glance, cry when I see them do something for others that just humbles the soul. I boast about them to others, whenever anyone will listen, and I thank God for his intervention and the surgeon and medical staff who helped me past my second surgery and onward to my third, whenever it may be. I guarantee, I will be in shape and I will get ready for it. If there is a record to be set with most open hearts, or longest life after, or feats accomplished after, I want to be there. I have to have goals, and when I reach one, I set another one. That is the way I coached and the way I live. My immediate goal I have now is to finish this book. The name of it is: "Life After Heart Surgery", so as I was writing, I was also living it and finally said: "It's time to stop and write the closing."

My Macker partner brother, Phil: Phil and I have been tight ever since I can remember; he has always had my back, from defending me at school to keep me out of scuffles, to saving me from drowning. He is such a caring man, I would take a bullet for him without hesitation and I know he would for me too.

He said this: When I first heard of Dave's first surgery, I was worried and nervous, because Dad died of a heart attack in 1975, and now my brother was having heart surgery. In 1989, I didn't know too much about bypass surgery, so I was worried, but I knew he was in great shape and very motivated. I knew he would do well, and he came through with flying colors. During the whole process I went from scared, to concerned, to relieved with his recovery. Dave's recovery time was incredible. I tried to tell him not to do things so fast, and to listen to the doctor, but Dave is Dave, and he did his own thing. The family prayed and supported each other, which helped everyone with their nerves.

When it was time for his second surgery, I was more worried. We knew he would need another surgery after about 10 years, and then all of a sudden, it was time. In my expectations of how Dave would do, once again, I knew he was in great shape, and was highly motivated, and that technology had really improved. I was so relieved when he was on the road to recovery, and then he was going back into surgery and I thought for the first time, that I was going to lose my brother. Throughout the whole process, I went from very nervous, prayed a lot, to relieved, to proud of Dave's steadiness, optimism and will power. His recovery was slower for Dave's expectation, and again I would keep telling him to listen to the doctor, and don't try to come back too fast.

Finally, I believe that attitude has a great influence on how things turn out, not just for the patient, but also for friends and family members. I'm so thankful to still have my brother here with us.

My big brother, Jeff, has always been 5 years older and into his age things, but our hearts were, are, and always will be bound to each other. Jeff is the writer, brainiac, of the brothers as you will see when you read his thoughts.

Big Bros' input begins'

Admittedly I had to regain my composure, set my pen down, reach for my handkerchief and dry the tears welling up; so that I could see to write. Before the ink hit this paper I was blowing my nose and still drying my eyes. Again the pen hit the table and I had to arise from my desk. I walked around for a minute or two and ended up looking out the window, gazing toward the heavens. I prayed for serenity, courage, and wisdom as I do on a daily basis; sometimes more than once. I expressed my gratitude for this day; that again, I was able to rise and find the face in the mirror was still smiling back at me. I re-captured my composure; after oneness with God, and my mind and heart started to spew verbiage.

Naturally my father's passing away, fifteen years prior, was still foremost on my mind when the news of Lil Bros' first surgery was imminent in the late 80's. This is where my mind went, and that was magnified even more so, and hit me really hard; after nearly three decades had transpired since dads' passing, and surgery number two became inevitable. I had my own moments of anxiety in the mid 90's when a Mitral Valve Prolapse provided me with a quick ambulance trip to Oakwood hospital in Dearborn Michigan. I never even knew the condition existed, which was masked by my ability to cope with stress, until the day I was physically assaulted on my job. That was the trigger that had never been pulled and then BANG, my heart was racing at about 160 beats per minute. The starting gun had been fired and I was hooked up to the EKG and an ensuing ride to the emergency room. I recall my thoughts that day and although I felt like a cat, who had just been chased up the tree by Marmaduke, my talons remained securely planted in the branches. I valued my job first and then thought about my chest. I thought best to not retaliate because I probably would be without an occupation, with zero tolerance allowed in the workplace. Now I was thinking about my wife, my children, and how things may turn out. Now I would concentrate on what was transpiring around me as I got wheeled in for the cath and the doctor explained what was going on. I felt no pain from the balloon which got the valve betwixt the left atrium and the ensuing chamber situated where it belonged. It wasn't until this time I even knew that the second chamber was screaming for the blood to flow and the valve was prohibiting what I had taken for granted. It would be mendacious on my part to deny that I was scared. Soon I was taking my meds and dealing with some stress management. It's truly a miracle the technology at our disposal in this millennium. Now faced with my brother's condition, the mere thought of losing him was enough to bring me to my knees. Although we may not have had a great deal of "one on one" time, what we shared was quality time and conversation when we could. We had a mutual understanding and although visits were short on time our relationship was long on love, admiration and respect. As motivated as my brother is, I knew, he would surmount the first surgery with flying colors. His competitive nature can be tantamounted only by defeat; which for David is NOT AN OPTION.

I felt different about his second surgery in 2002. I received a call on the eve of my 54th birthday that David was heading in again for open heart surgery. I recall getting off work on the 22nd at 4:30 AM and getting home for a five o'clock shower, anxious to trek to Lansing to see my Lil Bro. After a small breakfast I departed about six that morning from our Detroit metropolitan area and was headed north to Lansing for Ingham Memorial Hospital.

I arrived in Lansing at about 7:10 AM. I don't recall what time his surgery took place nor do I recollect the length of the procedure, but it was a long day and not the celebration I had anticipated for this date. He thought stents would be the call but open heart was the plan. My little brother was all psyched up and ready to get this done so he could return to coaching as the following week was the beginning of the Volleyball season. This procedure would be, "a walk in the park". David's' attitude and faith, being as positive as ever, made me feel a little more secure about the outcome. Knowing him as I do; he would most likely be lifting weights, climbing staircases, and swimming before long. This is his nature. If it's worth doing, it's worth overdoing, and he just won't allow himself to be held back. With this in mind, and his stable condition following the operation, we said our good-byes and I jumped back on the Interstate to head home knowing my athletic brother would be ready for competition before long and aspiring to new heights. I looked at it this way; it was like a re-birth and this would be his and my new mutual birthdays.

David was set to go home eight days later and then: I will never, ever, forget that phone call from Ronda on that day. The picture painted was a dismal one to say the least and I was not prepared. I was told "your brother is ready to go be with dad" "He has seen the light at the end of the tunnel". I was told that he had prepared himself for the after-life and to be at the right hand of God and be with our father. I was told his heart was so heavy; its' dead weight conceding to pain and agony and he was prepared for eternal bliss. These were not words I was accustomed to hearing and not words I wanted to hear about my youngest sibling. I was told of the excruciating pain in his chest, his shallow breathing and respiratory aids needed to get that valuable oxygen where it belonged, all the tubes and feeder tubes dispensing liquids and medication to his body. The body that I only knew as a world class physique was tied like an umbilical cord to monitors for watching his vital signs that became apparent to me there could be grave dangers ahead when I first saw him.

As I traversed that seventy two miles from door to door I wasn't really prepared for what I would see, but I certainly knew what I intended to say if David could even hear me. As I was heading north so were Mom and Herb who had done a 180 degree turn as they were headed to Florida at this time. The entire family was en-route almost simultaneously. As I entered the hospitals waiting area I gazed into the eyes of fear, anxiety, tears, wonderment, and a family unit once again knit in a common cause to support and pray for the best.

"Can I see my brother?" I asked. Being told it was okay I entered knowing from other family members not to expect any communication as it was next to impossible for him to respond. I still had things I desired to say. As my body entered his room and slid to his bedside, my tears again swelled and, I knew the message was clear. He looked real hopeless and yet peaceful if that was possible. I kissed him on his right cheek and then kissed him on his forehead. I placed the index finger of my right hand into his right palm and wrapped his digits around mine. I leaned over and whispered in his right ear. "David, I know you are prepared to be with our father and to be with our Lord; however I am a selfish man, as are others in this family, with the same angst, and it's not your time to go" "You have a loving wife, children who need your guiding hand, and a host of family here unwilling to allow you to succumb to this procedure." "We all love you and we need you desperately" "You will make it Lil Bro, just trust in God." It was not my imagination when I felt the grip around my finger tighten ever so slightly. Again my tears cascaded as I knew my warrior little brother would pull this one off and again cross the finish line a victor, as he had done over a dozen years prior. Now I did not feel completely hopeless about his condition because his vocabulary does not include DEFEAT. I felt like he had just passed the baton when I felt that slight finger squeeze and the race was on.

David's' motivation, his incessant training, his methodization, and his virtues of steadfastness have shown in his accomplishments through out his life. He has instilled the same in all of his prodigie's and the track record is clear; he has been a superb example in imparting his knowledge to all, regardless if you were an athlete, a student, a child, or to his family and friends. If one followed his game plan, and executed the same strategies and devotion he exemplifies, they certainly would be a winner or really close to the apex of the endeavors taken on. Whether it was a contest of athleticism or an earnestness for perfection David has translated this in all of his life's activities and proudly it shows.

I am very proud of you Lil Bro. Love Ya, Jeff

My friend Jack remembers thinking. How can this be happening to someone who looks so healthy? As a physical specimen, Dave appeared to be a picture of health. One thing I did know was that the hospital would not keep him long. He was out walking the streets in four days I think, and that didn't surprise me. Dave has more determination than any person I know. I knew he would come back quickly, but even I was surprised to see him out walking the streets for exercise as quickly as he was. I remember thinking that we all take heart surgery for granted anymore which is probably not wise, but I just knew that he would come out of all this and be the same old Dave.

I don't know all he did in his recovery phase, but I know, I've never seen anyone recover quicker than Dave, and get back to normal for him. Dave proved that if you stay in good shape and have determination, you can make this process go much better with a shorter recovery time. With Dave, it was never an attitude of "oh, poor me." It was always, here is a new challenge and I'm going to beat it. Amazing what a positive attitude can do for a person.

When he went in again for his second one, I thought. Here we go again, although with his heart and family history, it was no longer a surprise. I really didn't think it would be any different than the first, but I thought he might not bounce back quite as quickly. But I knew he'd be back to his old self, or kill himself trying! When he went back in for the surgery eight days later, then I really thought, this guy is human, and you can't take heart surgery for granted, and maybe his condition was worse than I thought. I was always hopeful for Dave throughout his surgeries. I have known some people who have given up the fight and the doctors could see no reason for them getting weaker, but they just plain refused to fight anymore. That is not Dave; I knew that would never happen with him. If there was one ounce of hope, he was determined to use it and *never* give up. When it took longer for Dave to bounce back from the second surgery, he seemed more like a normal person for that one. What Dave did show on both occasions, is that the mental part of it is way more important than most people think. Go in with a positive "I'm going to beat this thing" attitude, and recovery will be less painful and shorter.

My friend, Bob, of over 30 years said: I was not surprised, because I knew the men in Dave's family usually didn't live past their 50s, but I was concerned. I figured Dave would do well, because he caught the problem before any damage occurred from a heart attack. I felt like Dave was in good hands, and my wife and I did a lot of praying for him. I expected Dave to do well and he did fine and led an active life after the surgery. He had a positive attitude and recovered quickly. The second one happened so quickly, by the time I heard about it, he was experiencing difficulty and I thought that something had gone wrong, and this could be serious, so I felt helpless and could only pray for him. He got through it and recovery was slower, but his determination to beat this helped him along.

Kirk and Monti, great friends, write: We were very scared for him. I've never seen my husband cry, and the day we found out he was talking to Rhonda on the phone, and he just lost it. Dave is very close to him and it was painful news. We honestly didn't know what to expect. We knew that Dave is tough. We didn't know him when he had his first surgery. We prayed a lot for him.

I guess if we had expectations, then Dave would have exceeded them. When we saw him for the first time after surgery, we couldn't believe that he was doing so well and looked great too.

When we heard that he was going back into surgery, oh my God, we were scared poopless. We couldn't even imagine how Dave was feeling. It definitely confirmed to us that he is a strong person. Obviously, Dave was paying attention to his symptoms. During his ordeal, we kind of felt a little selfish, because we didn't want to lose a new and special friend. As far as Dave's recovery, he has his stuff together, and is very disciplined and focused. He is an amazing person.

I have had two very influential people in my life with the same first name, Richard, and my son now bears that as his middle name. One has passed away and this is from the other.

Dave and I have been close friends and lifting partners since 1983. Dave had always anticipated heart surgery because of his father's condition, so I know he wasn't surprised. I also knew what good shape he was in from lifting with him so much. I knew he was as "prepared" as he could be. As far as my expectations of how Dave would do with the surgery, I knew he'd do well. He keeps himself informed and plans ahead for everything, and as expected, he did very well. I do remember thinking how young he was to have the surgery, but again, he had anticipated it and it was no surprise to him. When he started into his training and recovery, I was impressed. I knew he would do great because we had spent a lot of time working out together and I know how determined he is and his ability to follow through on everything.

When he was headed in to have another surgery, I was thinking: "He just went through this" but in reality it was 13 years later. I knew that Dave anticipated another surgery and from experiencing the first one, I figured he would do fine again. I expected him to do well again because of his physical shape, he took pretty good care of himself, so even though he was older, I believed he'd recover well again. I think his second surgery was a little more difficult that I'd anticipated; once he went back in eight days later, I was concerned. That's when I got feelings that things weren't going to go as well as the first one. I prayed a lot that God would not take Dave yet, and prayed that Dave would heal and be able to recover and regain his active lifestyle. Once he was home and recovering and it was tougher than the first one, I also knew that if anyone could pull through this and get back to normal that Dave could.

## Now An Advocate Of Seeing Your Doctor

I have talked to many people who have had chest pains or some symptoms of heart trouble that I have convinced to go see their doctor and be checked. I met a lady on a train to Chicago and we talked and I learned that she had some problems and wasn't going to the doctor; due to some frustrating family turmoil that had taken its toll on her. The heart trouble seemed to come at the end of all the other problems and she was at the point of feeling, I just don't care what happens. I told her that I had gone through two surgeries and about the book I was writing. I talked to her about what kind of person she was after she described what she did for a living, which included many years of coaching swimmers. I said, you are an optimist, the cup is half full with you, not half empty, and when your kids swam and lost, you taught them how to win the next time. I told her that I expected her to make an appointment to be checked out when she got home from her trip. We exchanged emails and have written to each other since then.

I met a man in Jamaica who was from Canada and after speaking to his wife, she explained that he had troubles that he was ignoring, and I promised her to speak to him and try to convince him to check things out as well when they got home from their trip. I did speak to him, told him about my surgeries and the book and explained to him how others in his life want him around in their lives as long as possible and that he needed to go in and at least check things out. He listened and agreed that he probably should, but when I tried to get him to promise me to look into it, he said, "I'm not going to promise, but I'll think about it." That told me, my job is not done yet with him. We exchanged addresses and I will still be working on that one. If it is the next friend who finally convinces him to check it out, that's great, just as long as he does.

## Heart Transplant

I have a friend, Ron, whose story humbles mine, when he had a heart transplant. We have known each other for about 15 years but really never shared stories until I started this project of this book.

He was 48 years old in June of 1989, which is the same year of my first surgery, when he started into his struggle to stay alive. He was recovering from back surgery when he developed a cough, so he checked in with a doctor who said it was an upper respiratory infection. Well, it continued to get worse, and then, they thought it was pneumonia, so he went in and this time the doctor gave him a chest X-ray and the x-ray showed that his heart was twice its normal size. Another local doctor was consulted and he was off to Ingham where a left chest heart catheterization procedure took place. This test showed that there was no blockage and the lungs were good. But things still didn't feel good, so the next test took place at U of M Medical Center, with a heart catheterization of the left side of the heart and they took a biopsy and discovered idiopathic cardiomiopathy. This is a terrible virus/disease in the heart muscle that basically turns the heart muscle to mush. There is no cure; you must get a heart transplant before it causes your death.

At the time of all the tests, this healthy guy was 6'3" and 230 pounds, and was told that he would be put on the waiting list of a heart transplant. He was seventh on the list with his blood type and third on the list for a heart the size he needs, and it is a cruel fact, but 30% of the people on the list never receive a heart. When placed on the list, he was waiting for a heart based on his blood type and size, so that the replacement would be an adequate size for him. He was on the list for people between 200 and 230 pounds, and it could be a male or female donor. He had been working at the local university for 15 years in the custodial staff and was told to stop working immediately. He started to lose weight right away and months went by with him still on the waiting list, visiting the doctor every three weeks and getting worse and worse. By Thanksgiving, nearly six months later, he had lost 160 pounds and now weighed 160 (KJ note: that would have made him 320 originally, not 230), and was in a wheel chair. In his mind the end was near, so he asked the doctor if he could go out to the west coast and visit some family and bring his eight- and nine-year-old kids, so they could see the ocean and the west coast, and Disneyland. The doctor approved the trip and his son pushed the wheel chair that his Dad was in. During that Thanksgiving, all of his family thought this was the last time they would see him. His wife and kids, while scared and worried, held on to hope and faith that a heart would come through. He was glad to be able to provide that trip for his kids, and about a month later he went to the hospital on January 3$^{rd}$ of 1990. He says of himself at that time that he was relaxed and had an attitude of: If you want to take me now, I am ready. "My eyes were sunk in and I looked like death warmed over." He was admitted to the hospital, now moved onto the emergency list and was given not more than two more weeks to live without a transplant. On Jan 5$^{th}$ at 8:00 p.m., the hospital told him that they thought they had found a heart for him.

A 26-year-old male jogger was killed when hit by a car, and he was brought by land ambulance to the U of M Medical Center, where my friend was waiting. Then there was a final glitch, as the mother of the deceased was not interested in giving out parts of her son, so the anticipation was taken away as fast as they had it. The mother was still angry and sad that her son had been taken away and then a priest who was at the hospital talking to another heart transplant patient heard about the dilemma. The priest spoke to the mother and explained why he was there and how her son could benefit another's life with such an impact that could save and enhance someone else.

The mother agreed to many different organ donations and my friend was going to get his new heart. So on Jan 6th, he had his surgery. He was in intensive care until Jan 10th, when he was moved to an isolated room on the thoracic floor. The isolated room was a protection, in case of infection, and all nurses and visitors had to wear masks.

He would be the 122nd successful heart transplant by U of M Medical Center at that time.

He was in the UofM Medical Center for two weeks, and just three days after surgery, he was up and walking the circuit available to patients, even though he was connected to many tubes and the rolling tower with bags of medication. Once they let him, he was walking the circuit five and six times a day until they let him go home. Luckily, he didn't lose any more weight after surgery, and now at 6'3" and 160 pounds, the pole he was walking with was near the size of him, but he had a new chance on life, so weight didn't matter, and he started putting it back on right away. They also provided him with an exercise bike in his hospital room, which he used in addition to the walks in the hall. His last test at the hospital before being able to go home was to climb one flight of stairs, and as easy as that sounds, it isn't after surgery. By the end of the two weeks, he was ready and made it up the flight of stairs. Then the nurse said, OK, now go back down. He thought, all right, going down can't be that tough, but it was equally as hard. He made it and was released.

He came home from the hospital Jan 19th and was up to walking a mile a day and 10 minutes of bike per day.

Upon arrival home, he started his walks outside, even though it was winter in our state. His walks were longer at home, and he still went out two and three times per day. His parents stayed at his house with his wife and two kids, to help with whatever he may need. It was about three weeks later that he was doing very well and his parents went back to their home. He steadily gained his weight back and six months later, he was back to 200 pounds. That is a gain of about 7 pounds every month. He stayed out of work for a full year and at that time, he was 215 pounds.

They placed him on anti-rejection medication called

cyclosporine, as well as a steroid called prednisone. He also was required to come back in for tests quite often. He went in once a week for a while, then every two weeks, then every three weeks, then once a month, then every other month, then every three months, then four, and then twice a year. Each visit was for a small biopsy of his heart. They went through the neck with the catheter and took a small piece of his new heart and tested it for rejection. They had to stay on top of this test to make sure it wasn't being rejected. It has now been six to seven years since he has had to be tested, with no medication changes during that time, and he is now 65 years old.

Prior to going on the steroid, he had to go through psychological testing to determine his tolerance and temperament. They need to be cautious about prescribing steroids, because they can change a person's temperament. He jokingly claims he used to have a temper, but the medication was necessary and prescribed for his survival. One side effect of the medication is tremors, the shakes, in his hands, but in his positive spirit he joked that, "I make a heck of a martini, shaken, not stirred."

The medication cyclosporin was prescribed because his white blood cells were treating the new heart as a foreign substance in his body and treating it as something to fight off. As he tried to put it in laymen's terms, the anti-rejection medication makes his white blood cells drunk, and instead of rejecting the heart, it fools them not to reject it. A side effect of this med is that he is more susceptible to infections.. He has to be more careful with abrasions and any cuts, and some skin cancer and warts have occurred. He has had the same wart cut off five times, and many skin cancer spots taken off his hands. He also had skin cancer taken care of on his ear and they grafted some skin from his back, but the meds caused more growth to both areas than expected, so both areas bulged out more than expected by him or the doctors. Another effect that occurred from the meds is that the hair on his head is much thicker than it ever was before the transplant.

He returned to work one year later and while he felt healthy, there was something difficult about it. Others kept telling him, "You know, you don't have to work." This is when he learned from others that anyone with a heart transplant is considered "permanently disabled." This qualification allowed him to draw his retirement and

Social Security due to the disability. He has been a workaholic all his life and an adrenalin junkie and always worked hard, so this was a difficult decision to make. However, once he looked into it, and found that he was able to earn up to a certain amount and still be on his disability, this gave him and his family the stability they needed financially, and still allowed him to work and satisfy his need to do something.

He is careful about his diet, and he watches the cholesterol and fats intake.

He has given talks to many groups and classes about his transplant and the whole ordeal. He has spoken at Rotary Clubs, Lions Clubs, health classes in the local high school and middle school, some college classes and some nursing classes. His talks and information have been very valuable to many people.

He said he is so appreciative and owes this little town his life. The community pulled together with so many things to help him and his family. Remember that he was out of work for a long time while waiting for a heart and finances were tough. The family's medical insurance came out of his wife's check and didn't leave enough to cover the rest of the bills. The town took donations and showed up with cash for them. But it was done anonymously. The doorbell would ring and they would find an envelope with money in it, and no one there. People sponsored volleyball fundraiser tournaments and spaghetti dinners that raised money. Someone donated a beeper, so he could be contacted quicker when they found a heart for him. There was a time when he was afraid to leave the house, just in case the call came while he was out, but the beeper changed all that. "We didn't have cell phones yet," he said.

He was given a blue flasher light for the car to drive faster because he was three hours from the eventual surgery site. The local police were on standby with the intention of providing a police escort to a point where another town's police would take over and lead him to the surgery more quickly if needed. The newspaper ran pictures and announced other charitable events for benefits for finances. He has always been a hunter, and when he couldn't that year, somehow a deer walked into his garage, died, was gutted and processed, and the meat ended up in his freezer. His daughter dreamed of playing the clarinet, and suddenly there was one at the door and lessons to learn how to play it. His boy received the bike he dreamed about. The kids received clothes and many of these wonderful things occurred anonymously. People offered to care for the kids, the grass was cut, the garage was cleaned, a bank account was started at the local bank and people just donated money and deposited it. There were tickets sold for drawings for all kinds of donated wonderful prizes. His co-workers raised funds for him as well. ToysforTots contacted them and the family said, they had received enough, but appreciated their offer. He is certain that they would have lost their house without all that help.

It is now 17 years since his transplant and he has retired from his latest position at the school as a teacher's aid. He is so grateful to have been here to experience seeing his kids grow up, and he has been married to his wife for 31 years now. His daughter is now 29 years old, living and working in Alaska as a liaison for kids with families in turmoil. His son, now 27 years old, is in the Army National Guard. He has defended our country in Iraq and Dad is very proud of him, and glad he is now back home and safe.

I want to thank him for sharing with me, so I could bring some more information to you about heart success stories and "Life after Heart Surgery."

I met a second man while in Jamaica in February 2007, who was 82 years old and had just had a four-way bypass only three months before. He looked great. Not only did he not look 82, he didn't act it and it was only three months since his bypass. We were all in an all-inclusive resort and he had traveled from Virginia alone and was having a great time. Like me, he had cheated death more than once. He had gone down in a plane crash in WWII and survived, he had 17 years of chemotherapy for bone cancer and survived, and most recently his heart blockage and bypass surgery. He wasn't ready to give up by any stretch of the imagination, as a matter of fact, he was very interested in finding and having female companionship in his life.

It has been 5 1/2 years since my second open heart surgery and I have enjoyed many things that I could have missed.

My son who just turned 22 years of age is a college athlete and All-Patriot League Wide Receiver twice and graduate of Colgate

University in New York, and you can bet your bottom dollar that I didn't miss a game. I have been blessed to be able to see every game as I travel after him and watch him with pride in my heart. While I get excited when the team wins, I have to admit, I film him on every play with the zoom on and I follow his every move. I usually have to ask the person next to me what happened when Erik doesn't get the ball. If the pass is not to him, I can usually pick up on the play before it is done, but I am there to see and film my boy. When I get home after every game, I then go back through the film I just shot and place all the highlights on an annual highlights tape for Erik at the end of the season, and then transfer that to a DVD. I spend time with him after each game and then head back home and plan for the trip the next week.

I was able to watch my daughter's end of her junior season basketball and a lot of her games in her senior year also at Colgate University. Malissa graduated in 2004, just before Erik became a Raider. Malissa graduated with records in most 3-point shots made, total number of starts for Colgate and total number of minutes played for career. She also was named Patriot league tournament most valuable player. I was there for that tournament and many other games because of my surgeon's skills. Malissa went on to become the youngest Women's Basketball Director of Operations ever when she signed with Northwestern University, and I have visited her there and been to some of her games there as well, and now she has finished her Masters.

I was there to walk Crandall, my first born, down the aisle for her wedding and give a speech about her and her military husband, Jason, at their wedding reception. I was there for the birth of my grand daughter. I've been to their home in North Carolina and I owe all these things to the doctor who brought me back. I am so grateful to him and his staff. I was present at Erin's graduation from Kellog Community College, and watched her start her career as a Physical Therapy Assistant and become self-sufficient.

I recently have started a new job with a skilled craftsman labor support company, where I do interviewing and hiring of applicants and place them on job assignments. I have found that if you want something, then you just have to go for it.

## Listening To Your Body

This is so important. Many people, especially men do not go to see the Doctor when they should. They may feel a slight pain, or get dizzy occasionally, feel short of breath and pass it off as anything other than a clue that there is a problem with his heart. Men tend to work through pain, push through, and have been taught their whole life: "Not to wine", Don't be a baby, suck it up and so on. With this type of background, it is difficult to then say to yourself or your spouse, I think I need some help until it is so bad that by the time they go in, they may need the surgery already. I am now an advocate to others to get in there and check. I have always been very good about what I call. "Listen to your body" I have used it for myself and with all the athletes I have ever coached. I have talked to many people who have had chest pains or some symptoms of heart trouble who I have talked into to go see their Doctor and be checked.

## Second Divorce

Eventually, after 11 years, the varied backgrounds that my wife and I came from slowly deteriorated what we held dear. It's hard to pinpoint when it was that we crossed the line of really not having an interest in the others interests, concerns and beliefs, but it happened and it was just a matter of time before we knew that we were not meant for each other. I have learned a lot about hearts during my life and surgeries and subsequent recoveries, and stress is a huge component in heart problems. The stress has been reduced and it was a necessary concern that had to be addressed.

## Plan B For Income

I continue with my MLM, home based business work. I have become a Vice President in the company and my site is www.savepetro.mybpi.com

The program is lucrative and the product is amazing. In these days and soaring prices in gas and diesel fuel, I have found a product that actually increases Miles per gallon in any vehicle. The product has been tested and proven to work by the EPA recognized Wallace Labs Inc., a group who has been testing these products since 1984. I can be contacted about this great product at upyourmpg@yahoo.com or at my website. This is a great way to make an extra income for anyone, and especially heart patients because it affords you the flexibility to work as much as you want, and when you do work, all you are doing is talking to people, sharing a product that everybody needs and wants when you tell them about it.. How easy is that? If you have learned anything about me, it is that I believe in The Pure, The Positive, and The Powerful. I would not be working and promoting this product unless it worked.

## Closing

I have had great difficulty in knowing if this book is finished, or complete, and I finally decided that it will never be finished in my mind, as it is about: "Life After Heart Surgery", and as long as there is time after the surgery, it is ongoing. I have enjoyed going down memory lane with the idea that it may help someone in some way. If you or someone in your family, or a friend faces heart surgery,. God bless them and you as you head into this adventure, and I pray that all goes as well with your surgery as it has with mine.

**I have to say that the love and support of my family, and prayer have been so strong that it has helped me at every step of the way, and no words can describe any way to thank them enough. My parents are still there for me and they are in their 80's. My kids are so supportive and I am so proud of the mature adults that they have become. My brothers, even though we are separated by miles in geography and our busy lives, the heartfelt bond with them is solid as it can be. Finally, my friends who have been behind me all the way. God Bless you all.**

Printed in the United States
128728LV00002B/87/P